About the Author

Kathryn Marsden is a nutritionist who, for many years, worked in full-time clinical practice in the UK. She is probably best known as the author of the bestselling books *The Complete Book of Food Combining* and *Good Gut Healing*, and she has also contributed regularly to a wide range of media including national and local press, magazines, television and radio. Her books and articles are enjoyed by many for the lighthearted, humorous and frank way she describes the workings of the digestive system.

In 2003, Kathryn gave up her nutrition work in order to pursue other interests in her intended semi-retirement. However, a Spanish GP and a leading hospital consultant persuaded her to return. As a result, much of her time is now taken up holding voluntary nutrition clinics in a busy doctor's practice where she is the dietary adviser. She believes that excellent nutrition is incredibly powerful: 'If I can use my work as a writer and as a practitioner to change for the better the way people look after themselves (and in particular, their forgotten intestines), and if because of it their health improves or the risk of illness is lessened, then that makes me very happy indeed.'

KATHRYN MARSDEN

Good
GutBugs

How the healing power of probiotics can
transform your health

piatkus

For Trish Dicksee

Long may the energy of bright red running shoes permeate your household and the turquoise of wisdom animate your spirit.

PIATKUS

First published in Great Britain in 2010 by Piatkus
Copyright © Kathryn Marsden 2010

The moral right of the author has been asserted

A CIP catalogue record for this book
is available from the British Library

ISBN 978-0-7499-4044-7

Typeset in Meridien by Action Publishing Technology Ltd, Gloucester
Printed and bound in Great Britain by MPG Books, Bodmin, Cornwall

Papers used by Piatkus are natural, renewable and recyclable
products sourced from well-managed forests and certified
in accordance with the rules of the Forest Stewardship Council.

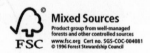

Mixed Sources
Product group from well-managed
forests and other controlled sources
www.fsc.org Cert no. SGS-COC-004081
© 1996 Forest Stewardship Council
FSC

Piatkus
An imprint of
Little, Brown Book Group
100 Victoria Embankment
London EC4Y 0DY

An Hachette UK Company
www.hachette.co.uk

www.piatkus.co.uk

WANTED

GOOD GUT BUG

FOR CHALLENGING POSITION AS:

BENEFICIAL MICROBE

WORK INVOLVES:

- CONTROLLING HARMFUL BACTERIA
- STRENGTHENING NATURAL DEFENCES
- REDUCING THE RISK OF BOWEL DISORDERS
- HELPING TO PREVENT INFECTIONS
- PROMOTING DIGESTION
- AIDING THE ABSORPTION OF NUTRIENTS FROM FOOD
- IMPROVING INTESTINAL MICROBIAL BALANCE
- COOLING INFLAMMATION
  AND
- SUPPORTING THE IMMUNE SYSTEM

Applicant should be adaptable, friendly and not easily intimidated

Must be able to work on own initiative as well as part of a team

Long hours, no holidays

Balanced attitude essential

Notes for Readers

Kathryn's views are completely independent. She is not employed by any pharmaceutical company, supplement supplier or food producer, nor is she persuaded in any way, financially or otherwise, to recommend particular products or services.

The information that Kathryn includes in all her books has been accumulated from published journals, meetings and discussions with a number of different practitioners, medical and surgical consultants and other experts, and from her own personal research, training and experience in practice.

The guidelines suggested in *Good Gut Bugs* are not intended to be prescriptive, nor are they an attempt to diagnose or treat any specific condition. Kathryn always emphasises that no one should stop taking their prescribed medication without first talking to their GP or specialist. Certain medicines are essential for life, but longer than necessary use of others or of particular combinations of drugs could cause health problems due to side effects, nutrient deficiencies and/or interactions. Kathryn therefore also recommends that patients keep a careful note of all drugs and ask for a regular medical review of repeat prescriptions. She is unable to comment on specific case histories or to reply individually to correspondence. However, she is always delighted to hear from readers and does read every letter.

Contents

Part Two: Probiotic Support for Particular Problems

Part Three: Supplements and Safety

Foreword by
Dr Vicente Mera Sánchez

The world is full of microbes, and so are people's bodies (the skin, gut and natural orifices act as reservoirs of bacteria). We already know that 'friendly' bacteria are vital both to the proper development of the immune system as well as assisting the digestion and absorption of food and nutrients. On the other hand, an overgrowth of 'unfriendly' disease-causing bacteria can upset this critical balance. Experts are exploring how probiotics and prebiotics could halt these pathogens in their tracks and suppress their growth and activity. In particular they are studying digestive conditions, namely infectious diarrhoea, irritable bowel syndrome, inflammatory bowel disease, ulcers and chronic stomach inflammation due to *Helicobacter pylori*, and also tooth decay and periodontal disease, urinary, vaginal and respiratory infections. Allergy and eczema recurrences are among the non-infectious diseases where probiotics have also shown themselves to be beneficial.

Probiotics have been the treatment of choice for many nutrition-oriented practitioners for many years. Yet, despite considerable research and huge interest in probiotics and prebiotics, neither is currently considered to be part of the arsenal of conventional medicine. Conventional and complementary medicine are both separated and joined by a fence. Nowadays, to cross the interconnecting gate from one side to another, a huge body of evidence regarding benefits and risks is mandatory. Kathryn Marsden is a nutrition expert with the uncommon virtue of being thorough in her work and balanced in her approach. This book, *Good Gut Bugs*, gives us the keys to open the gate between these two branches of medicine.

Dr Vicente Mera Sánchez
Hospital Clinica Benidorm, Spain

Foreword by Dr Jen W. Tan

It wasn't so long ago that the very idea of anyone having bacteria in their bowels was considered to be a rather bizarre concept, never mind that these bacteria could be good or bad for you. Think of the associations: bowels and faeces; bacteria and dirt. No wonder gut bacteria have had a rather Cinderella existence. Now, however, both probiotics and prebiotics are better understood and are beginning to be accepted by the medical profession.

Indeed, the science of probiotics and prebiotics has developed at an astonishing rate over the past 10 to 15 years. We now know that the impact of having the right type of bacteria existing within a conducive internal gut environment has profound and far-reaching effects on our health. Science has surprised us by showing that other organ systems, including the immune system, are influenced by the type of friends we have in our gut.

In this excellent book, Kathryn Marsden describes the role of gut bacteria in a clear and concise manner, balancing what is now accepted orthodoxy with empirical experience already familiar to many of those working in the field of complementary medicine. It has to be recommended to anyone seeking to better understand how this area of emerging science can be used to improve and maintain health.

Dr Jen W. Tan MB BS

Acknowledgements and Thanks

To Dr Vicente Mera for the back up of his vast medical knowledge and additional technical input, for always listening to my ideas and for reading every word – which I know he did.

To Dr Jen Tan for his foreword and always helpful comments.

To Dr Luis Cebrian for checking large chunks of the manuscript, and a special thank you for twisting my arm to join his clinic team. I've loved every minute.

To Dr Jeremy Burton in New Zealand for his endless patience in answering my many emails and for his extremely helpful suggestions and additions.

To Dr Mary Ellen Sanders in the US for helping me through the minefield of labelling legislation and for her guidance and corrections to the chapter on choosing probiotic supplements.

To Carol Hicks RGN, the best of nurses, for checking the medical minutiae and for her nursing knowledge.

To Gillian Hamer, for her nutritional and science expertise and for the encouragement, common sense and wise counsel given so generously throughout this project.

To Colette Harris – fellow bookworm and loyal correspondent – for her experienced editor's eye, her always excellent suggestions and for her contributions to the cover copy.

To Sue McGarrigle for contributing some of the technical material and for checking certain technical aspects of the work. The idea for this book was hers, not mine.

To dearest Georgina, copywriter par excellence, for doing so much proofing for me when she has so little free time.

And last but never ever least, always and forever, to Richard, my husband, dearest friend in all the world and bedrock of my life, I will love you for the rest of my life, beyond it and back again.

Introduction

If I told you that something you can't even see with the naked eye – something that lives naturally in the murky depths of your digestive system – could be a major factor in determining the difference between health and disease, and that paying it a bit more attention could significantly alter the odds against getting sick, I'd like to bet that you'd be interested. Forget expensive drugs and extreme diets; there are no excessive claims or empty promises here. This has to do with amazing research and the work of some of the world's leading scientists into the extraordinary goings-on in our intestines. To be specific, they're studying – look away now if you're squeamish – bacteria! If it makes you feel any better, be comforted by the fact that the particular bacteria in question are of the especially helpful and nice variety.

When someone mentions bacteria, most people will think of germs or infectious illness. But talk about beneficial bacteria and I imagine nearly everyone will either picture a pot of yoghurt or at least make some kind of connection to the digestive system. The idea that fermented foods (those that are made as a result of bacterial changes), such as yoghurt, might be healthy for humans is nothing new. The use of fermentation as a way of preparing and preserving food is steeped in ancient traditions and, long before anyone knew anything about good gut bugs, so-called primitive peoples had already worked out for themselves that cultured dairy foods such as soured milks and yoghurts were somehow beneficial. Thanks to modern research, we now know that the reason why fermented foods are good for us is because they contain beneficial strains of 'live culture'. These days, we have come to know these live cultures by another name: PROBIOTICS.

Although they've been tagged 'guardian angels of the gut', scientific studies strongly suggest that there's far more to probiotics than merely an ability to address digestive disorders. They're important to other areas of the body too.

So how does all this affect you?

First of all, there's no longer any doubt that maintaining the right level of beneficial bacteria in our intestines is incredibly important to the health of every human. That's because these mysterious microflora protect us from a whole host of nasty diseases. Without at least some 'good guys', we'd be very sick indeed and, without any at all, would soon die. In fact, I wonder how many of us realise just how much of our health is controlled by good gut bugs and just how much can go wrong as a result of the lack of them?

I'll always be grateful that I was starting my nutrition studies at a time when probiotics were first beginning to be recognised as essential to health. Can that be nearly 25 years ago? Even though probiotic use was very limited at the time, I certainly felt that we were learning about something valuable, something essential for everyone's health, something exciting. But most of the GPs I spoke to at the time had little or no information about these beneficial bugs. Even a few who had heard about friendly flora, mostly from well-informed patients, didn't think they were significant or worth bothering with. A handful of medics showed a real interest in the work I was doing, but some were actively hostile. I can remember one doctor dismissing the idea of good gut bugs as a nonsense waste of time, and a second saying that they were of no consequence whatsoever. 'Yet another example of alternative claptrap,' was the scathing opinion I shall never forget from a consultant gastro-enterologist who grudgingly granted me a five-minute audience. And while his sidekick registrar conceded that friendly bacteria 'might have something', he felt that they would probably always remain the province of fringe medicine or be limited to a few ancient tribes. I'd love to ask them all what they think now.

Even today, I think it would be fair to say that although probiotic research is creating huge interest among the scientific community and has been an important part of alternative therapy for many years, it has never really tickled the fancy of mainstream medicine. But things are changing.

The new buzz word

Now, bang up-to-date, the word 'probiotic' is part of everyday advertising and an ingredient in a whole range of yoghurts, yoghurt-type drinks (sometimes known as probiotic shots), milkshakes, smoothies, cereals, desserts, snacks, baby formula and, of course, supplements. Aside from foods, powders and pills, scientists are developing specific probiotics to prevent cavities, probiotic lozenges for sore throats, probiotic nasal sprays, probiotics to guard against ear infections, and probiotic deodorant sticks that deal with the bacteria that cause body odour. They're talking about probiotic vaccines to treat inflammatory diseases and even probiotic cleaning products for the home. The search is also on for a probiotic solution to improve immunity against bacterial meningitis. You may not have realised it before now, but the 'P' word is well on its way to becoming a multibillion dollar/euro/sterling industry. And yet, even though it looks as if all of this confirms for sure that probiotics are good for our health, the real purpose of these beneficial bacteria is still a mystery to most of us.

Unfortunately, as almost always happens with something new, the real science is being exaggerated by commercialism with all kinds of claims being made for beneficial bacteria that simply aren't true. Even a cursory casting across the worldwide Web through only a handful of the (last time I looked) 2,750,000 search options could leave you with the impression that probiotics are the panacea for all ills – the ultimate magic bullet. However, much of the praise is commercially driven by the companies who sell the products. Some seem happy to promise good results without giving any kind of scientific back-up or referenced documents but others, who are more enlightened, do provide valuable information about any relevant research.

On the other side of the coin are those who would have us believe that probiotics should be renamed 'conbiotics' and are nothing more than some kind of snake oil for the new millennium. Like everything else in life, the truth lies somewhere in between. Probiotics are not a cure-all and not all types are suitable for all people but, as scientific studies are showing repeatedly, they are without a doubt helpful for a wide range of health problems. I don't believe that it's an over-exaggeration to suggest that, in terms of health benefits and therapeutic activity, probiotics (especially when they are used in conjunction with important food substances known as prebiotics) could be to the 21st century what the good side of antibiotics were to the 20th.

Even so, at this stage of the game, the whole thing can seem like a bit of a minefield.

Getting to grips with it all

Apart from the scientists involved in the research, the micro-biologists who work with leading manufacturers and perhaps a few nutrition-oriented practitioners, it's hard for most people to know whether a particular product or food is going to be helpful or not. What's hype and what's authentic? Is that probiotic pill a good one? Is that probiotic yoghurt really 'live'? Do those probiotic sup-cplements genuinely contain enough active ingredients? Is it all just down to clever advertising? What does that label mean? You might even end up asking, 'Do I really need them?'

Although it's highly likely, in my view, that almost every single one of us would benefit from having more friendly flora in our systems, the sad fact is that most people are seriously deficient in the good-gut-bug department. So, what if I suggested that the right probiotics – together with their prebiotic partners – might have the power to alleviate or treat a whole range of health problems and could perhaps prevent serious illness?

Controlled clinical trials, laboratory studies and empirical evidence from clinical practice all strongly suggest an important role for probiotics in human health. A quick shimmy down this list should give you a really good idea of the potential power of probiotics and why they're being accepted more and more as essential to our health; for example, it's already been shown that they may have a role to play in:

- Reducing the risk of urinary infections.
- Helping heal vaginal infections and clearing up discharge.

- Lessening the side effects caused by antibiotics.
- Cutting the chances of going down with infective or travellers' diarrhoea.
- Treating children with diarrhoea.
- Lowering cholesterol.
- Helping reduce the symptoms of *C. difficile* colitis.
- Reducing the duration of colds and respiratory infections.
- Controlling and limiting the growth of unwanted bacteria, yeasts and parasites.
- Easing childhood eczema.
- Helping protect against tooth decay.
- Improving the transit time of food through the gut.
- Treating constipation.
- Easing the symptoms associated with IBS.
- Increasing resistance to infection.
- Settling disturbed digestion and easing bloating, burping and gas.
- Improving resistance to allergies whether from food, chemicals or the environment.

That's not all. This is just the beginning ...

Great ways forward

Now, researchers are getting very excited about the possibility that probiotics might have anti-carcinogenic, anti-mutagenic and anti-allergic actions and could hold an important key to serious conditions such as bowel cancer, asthma, Crohn's disease, ulcerative colitis, type-1 diabetes, fibromyalgia and chronic fatigue syndrome.

There's also huge interest in preliminary research suggesting that probiotics might even be able to enhance weight loss. Given the current figures on the number of people who are seriously overweight or dangerously obese and the acknowledged epidemic of type-2 diabetes and other weight-related diseases, this can only be good news.

Adding the right kind of probiotics to a good diet is one of the best health investments a person can make. While the majority of research focuses on specific health problems, there are also a number of studies demonstrating that probiotics have the power to keep healthy people healthy by lessening the likelihood of catching a cold or respiratory infection, reducing absence from work and increasing the number of illness-free days.

What also interests me is the potential of probiotics – and their prebiotic team-mates – to significantly decrease health-care costs, not only through their use in therapeutic medicine but also because of their power as a preventive. And not just here, but in the developing world, too. Perhaps probiotics could play a future significant role in the health of people, especially of children, in poor countries by helping to treat or reduce the risk of diarrhoeal illnesses that, without access to hospital care, are so often killers. It's also been suggested that probiotics could provide additional protection for aid workers and those who travel from relatively safe industrialised countries into more remote bacteria-risky areas of the globe.

The proof of practice

I need no persuading. I've been using probiotics in practice for the best part of two decades now as part of a range of treatment programmes and have seen some truly excellent results, including alleviating some conditions that had responded to no other treatment.

This book will show you, too, how your health can profit from probiotics. I'll be telling you about a whole stack of common conditions that might benefit from what we've come to think of as friendly flora. I'll also look at why things go wrong, the problems that can be caused by an overgrowth of bad bacteria, and how simple dietary changes and the healing properties of probiotics and prebiotics can help so much towards redressing the balance. Come on in.

What's between the pages?

Good Gut Bugs is divided into three parts:

Part One

I'll be giving you the goods on what probiotics really are, what makes them happy, what upsets and damages them and what you can do to create the right environment in your intestines to make it the perfect place for good gut bugs to thrive. We'll take a glance at the research behind beneficial bacteria and see how this new drug-free approach can be of benefit to so many different conditions. You'll read about the supportive power of probiotics, discover what they can do for you and for your long-term health and how the right kind of prebiotic diet is essential for their survival.

Before you start Part One, complete the questionnaire, Your Personal Health Map, on page 11. It should make you think about your current health status and what you can do to improve it. In the Good Gut Upgrade (Chapter 2), you'll be able to get into the diet side of things right away with plenty of healthy-eating advice.

Part One also covers a down-to-earth journey through the digestive system (Chapter 3) and all you need to know about *pre*biotics (Chapter 4), as well as a whole new and very important angle on fibre (Chapter 6).

There's an in-depth look at the upsides and downsides of antibiotics in Chapter 7 and the scary facts about superbugs in Chapter 8. Finally, the end of Part One is especially for those of you who lead such manic lives that sitting down and reading a whole book is generally out of the question. Chapter 9 contains an emergency action plan, which I've called If You Do Nothing Else . . .

Part Two

In Part Two we'll get down to some specifics and talk about how incorporating probiotics – and their prebiotic partners – into the diet can make a difference to a whole range of health problems. I've tended to concentrate on the conditions that have, so far, been the subject of most research. These include allergies, poor immunity, cholesterol, inflammatory bowel disease (IBD), irritable bowel syndrome (IBS), diarrhoea, constipation, colon cancer, lactose intolerance, *Helicobacter pylori* infection and urogenital health including bacterial vaginosis, cystitis and thrush. I'll also be looking at poor digestion and other gut disorders, repeated colds and respiratory infections, body odour and bad breath, all' of which can be made worse by low levels of friendly flora in the system. Kicking off Part Two is a very important description of a condition known as dysbiosis, included first because it can be the mystery trigger for a long list of other health problems.

Part Three

In Part Three I'll talk about things like supplements and safety. There's information on probiotic pills, capsules, powders and foods, how to choose good products, what to avoid, what to take, when to take them, and how much.

I've also included some Frequently Asked Questions and a Resources section to help you find reliable suppliers.

I hope you find the book informative and enjoyable. In the meantime, please breathe deeply, chew thoroughly and smile more, although not necessarily in that order or all at the same time.

Wishing you the best of better health.

Kathryn Marsden

What do the symbols mean?

Every now and then, throughout *Good Gut Bugs*, you'll come across some symbols. Here's what they mean:

For more info
If you see a sign like this, it's directing you to a subject in another part of the book that might be especially relevant.

Jargon buster

When you come across a word with the letters [JB] alongside it, there'll be a Jargon Buster box somewhere nearby.

Snippet
The scissor sign separates out snippets of information that I thought you might find interesting or fun.

Very important point
Where you see an exclamation mark, this indicates a very important point that I think is worth emphasising.

Did you know?
Boxes with bites of info that should help to add to your understanding.

In more detail . . .
You'll still get a really good idea of the benefits of probiotics if you decide to skip these sections, but reading them may help you to broaden your insight into a particular condition, treatment or related subject. And because *Good Gut Bugs* may also be of interest to practitioners and other health professionals, a more detailed explanation of some areas might be helpful.

Take care
An occasional 'hand' indicates something that you should be wary of or just be aware of.

How Do You Know if You Need Probiotics?

'The balance of nature is obvious most often when it is disturbed '

John Postgate, Emeritus Professor of Microbiology at
the University of Sussex, from his book *Microbes and Man*
(Cambridge University Press, 2000)

Before you read any further, find out whether you need probiotics by completing the following questionnaire. This will give you your Personal Health Map. In the questionnaire you'll find some boxes to fill in, which should help you to assess your current health status.

First, look through the symptoms and situations, and mark the appropriate spaces with the letters A, B, C or D as indicated; for example:

If you've never, or hardly ever, had acid indigestion, as in question 1, then mark the space in the first column with an A. (Never or hardly ever would mean maybe only once or twice during your lifetime.)

If you've suffered occasionally with bloating, as in question 2, perhaps no more than once every five years, then mark the space in the second column with a B.

If you suffer from constipation several times a year, as in question 7, then mark the space in the third column with a C. (If it's most of the time, then the fourth column, D, is the box for you.)

Complete one box in each section only

Next, copy the letter from your completed line into the Score Totals column on the right of each chart before moving on to the next question. Think carefully before you mark each box and be honest with your answers. If you think you don't fit into any particular box, then just go for the nearest option.

Questionnaire: Your Personal Health Map

Your general health

DO YOU SUFFER FROM?	Never or hardly ever If this applies to you, mark the box with an A	Only a few times during my life If this applies to you, mark the box with a B	Several times a year If this applies to you, mark the box with a C	Most or all the time or almost every day If this applies to you, mark the box with a D	Score totals
Acid indigestion (heartburn) or acid reflux					
Bloating					
Bad breath (halitosis)					
Body odour					
Burping or belching					
Colds					
Constipation					
Diarrhoea					
Difficulty digesting milk					
Food cravings					

DO YOU SUFFER FROM?	Never or hardly ever If this applies to you, mark the box with an A	Only a few times during my life If this applies to you, mark the box with a B	Several times a year If this applies to you, mark the box with a C	Most or all the time or almost every day If this applies to you, mark the box with a D	Score totals
Fungal infections of the mouth, nails or feet					
Hiatus hernia					
Hormonal disturbance such as PMS or hot flushes					
Itchy nose					
Itchy bum					
Irritable Bowel Syndrome (IBS)					
Loud gurgling in the belly					
Passing wind					
Respiratory allergies such as hay fever or to moulds, house dust, etc					
Sensitivity to any food					
Stinky poo					
Stomach pain					
Thrush					
Tummy bugs					
Digestive ulcers					
Urinary infections					
Vaginal discharge					

Family health history

WHICH OF THESE APPLIES TO YOU OR YOUR FAMILY?	If you suffer from any of these conditions NOW, mark the relevant box with a D. If not, leave blank	If you have a family history of any of these conditions, mark the relevant box with a C. If not, leave blank	Score totals
Allergies	D		D
Asthma as a child			
Asthma as an adult			
Circulatory problems			
Coeliac disease	D		D
Crohn's disease			
Diabetes	D	C	D
Eczema as a child			
Eczema as an adult			
Heart disease			
Helicobacter pylori (ulcers)			
High blood pressure			
High cholesterol			
Psoriasis			
Rheumatoid arthritis			
Thrombosis			
Ulcerative colitis			

Going to the doctor

HOW OFTEN DO YOU GO TO THE DOCTOR?	I'm never ill. I rarely go except for screening or routine check-ups	Once a year at the most	Quite often	Regularly, because I have a long-term health problem	Score total
	Mark the box with an A	Mark the box with a B	Mark the box with a C	Mark the box with a D	

Going to the dentist

HOW OFTEN DO YOU GO TO THE DENTIST?	Just for routine check-ups, but I hardly ever need treatment	Just for routine check-ups and the occasional filling	Every time I go I seem to need treatment	I never go to the dentist, because I can't afford it/ I'm too afraid/I just don't bother	Score total
	Mark the box with an A	Mark the box with a B	Mark the box with a C	Mark the box with a D	
	A		C		A

The truth about your diet

NOW'S THE TIME TO BE HONEST ABOUT YOUR EATING HABITS		Enter A, B, C or D	Score totals
I really care about what I eat and do everything I can to avoid unhealthy foods.	If this sounds like you, award yourself an A		
I do try to eat healthily, but I don't eat as much fibre or as many fresh fruits and vegetables as I should.	Not too bad, but perhaps you could try harder. Enter B	B	B
There never seems to be enough time to eat healthily. I try hard but never seem to quite get there.	Oops! Give yourself a C		
I know my diet is terrible. I eat too much junk and rely most of the time on packets, cans and/or takeaways.	Sorry, a definite D here		

Your antibiotic history

HOW OFTEN HAVE YOU NEEDED TO TAKE ANTIBIOTICS OVER THE PAST 15 YEARS?	Never	Once a year	I always seem to be on them for something	I have a health condition which means I have to take antibiotics most of the time	Score total
	Mark the box with an A	Mark the box with a B	I'd like to say C, but D is nearer the mark	Mark the box with a D	
		B			B

Other medicines

WHAT ABOUT OTHER MEDICINES?	If the answer is yes, mark the box with a D	If the answer is no, mark the box with an A	Score total
Do you take any kind of regular daily medication such as statins, steroids, inhalers or acid-suppressing drugs?		A	A

Now that you've finished, look back over each chart to see which letters you used the most. Now check the comments section below.

How did you do?

Mostly As

If you answered mostly As, then give yourself a special award. You seem to be in good shape and doing what you can to stay that way. So, is there any need for you to take probiotics or to add more prebiotic foods to your diet? I would if I were you. I've completed these charts several times over the years just to keep a check on my own health. So far, I've been lucky to have answered A for nearly every column, but that doesn't stop me topping up with probiotics and making sure that prebiotics are a significant part of my diet. Why not look upon both probiotics and prebiotics as good health insurance?

Mostly Bs

If your results are mostly Bs, then I'd guess you might say your health isn't too bad, but perhaps it could be better? Making improvements now could help prevent serious problems later on. At the very least read the Good Gut Upgrade (page 35), If You Do Nothing Else (page 141) and Probiotic Supplements (page 265).

Mostly Cs

So you scored mostly Cs? Would I be right in suggesting that your health problems are beginning to get in the way of your enjoyment of life? Perhaps this is the time to start making a few changes? We know from research done so far that there may be a link between low levels of good gut bugs and many of the conditions listed in the questionnaire. This doesn't mean that probiotics are a complete answer to every illness, but evidence is emerging that they can be helpful in easing symptoms, reducing the risk of side effects from some drugs and lessening the likelihood of certain diseases occurring in the first place. Part Two of *Good Gut Bugs*, which begins on page 147, may be relevant to you, because it covers a range of common complaints that could be helped by probiotics. While you're working through the rest of the book, perhaps you could introduce some of the advice in the Good Gut Upgrade (page 35).

Mostly Ds

If your answers were mostly Ds, then that could mean D for Danger or D for Dysbiosis (the condition described on page 149), especially if you leave the situation as it is and don't do anything about it. Lots of Ds could also suggest that your resistance to illness isn't as good as it could be, and could it also be that you're not so well at the moment? Perhaps you're having to take one or more different medications, too? Probiotics, in conjunction with an improved diet, could give you that extra boost and, at the same time, might ease some of your symptoms and side effects. Why not make a start right now? Most of this book is important for you but, in particular, please read the chapters on Dysbiosis (page 149), Prebiotics (page 68), Antibiotics (page 105) and the all-important Good Gut Upgrade which begins on page 35.

Important note

When you're not feeling so good, it can sometimes be difficult to know if the discomfort you're experiencing is something that's harmless and what doctors call self-limiting (in other words, it'll go away on its own and you'll be fine) or a problem you should be concerned about. This questionnaire is not attempting to diagnose any particular condition, but it might guide you towards your best course of action. If you've been under par for some time or are suffering persistent discomfort, and nothing you do seems to help, especially if you have any pain or shortness of breath, are plagued by repeated infections or are constipated, then please go to see your GP or specialist.

Part One

Getting the Balance Right

1.

What Exactly are Probiotics?

‘Remember that just because you're not sick it doesn't mean you're healthy. ’

Author unknown

As far as we know, the term 'probiotics' originally turned up in medical literature back in 1953, when it was coined to explain organic and inorganic supplements 'necessary to restore health to patients suffering a form of malnutrition resulting from eating too much highly refined food'. Too much highly refined food in 1953? Considering that this was still at the point where some countries were only just coming to the end of food rationing resulting from the Second World War, such a comment might have been seen as pretty advanced thinking for its time. But it was 1974 before the word was first used to explain the effect that helpful bacteria can have in improving the health of the intestines.

Today, probiotics are described officially by the Food and Agriculture Organization of the United Nations (FAO) and World Health Organization (WHO) as 'live microorganisms that, when administered in adequate amounts, confer a health benefit to the host'. The 'host', by the way, is you or me, which means that these microbes have to be shown through human studies to be of benefit to human health.

To be absolutely accurate, a 'probiotic' is a therapeutic agent that's supplemented from outside the body in the form of a food substance, tablets, capsules or powder. But the word 'probiotic' has become so synonymous with 'friendly flora' that it's often applied as an all-encompassing term (even though that's not quite correct) to describe all kinds of beneficial bacteria – whether these are the ones that already live inside us or the ones we take in food or supplements.

Perhaps a better way to think of probiotic bacteria is as commuters or straphangers, workers who travel through the gut to a particular destination in order to support the resident bacteria who make up the main gut inhabitants. Probably the easiest way to get it straight is to remember that the probiotic supplements we swallow are *supplementing* the health not only of our intestines but also of the whole body.

Did you know?
The word 'probiotic' is usually taken to mean 'for life' (from the Greek *Pro* = for (promoting), *biotic* = life). I like to think of probiotics as being 'for the encouragement of life'. It certainly seems to be the case that if they're present in the body in sufficient numbers, they're capable of providing health benefits that go way beyond basic healthy eating.

Micro what?

When scientists and medical researchers talk about those friendly bacteria that occur naturally within the body, you usually hear them say things like 'live microbial organisms' or, occasionally, 'beneficial intestinal flora'. Sometimes they talk about 'microbes' although this also includes other microscopic life such as mould spores, viruses and protozoa. Or they might refer to bacteria as 'microflora' or – a less familiar word, but a more correct term – 'microbiota'. It all means pretty much the same thing. As far as this book is concerned – and to keep things simple – just think of them as good gut bugs.

Antibiotic, probiotic – what's the difference?

People often ask if it's right to say that antibiotics are the opposite of probiotics – and vice versa. For sure, the actual words themselves are antonyms (opposite to each other in their meaning). When it comes to their natural behaviour, probiotics support life, but antibiotics – because they're used to halt the growth of bacteria – do the opposite, and can therefore be considered as the 'destroyers' of tiny living organisms. It's also true to say that probiotics have a natural antibiotic action of their own in that they're capable of dealing with small numbers of bad bacteria. It's only when parts of the body become overrun with bad guys that antibiotic drugs become necessary.

And what about the Latin?

Those long names, such as *Lactobacillus acidophilus* or *Bifidobacterium bifidum*, that you see written on the sides of certain food products, such as yoghurt, are some of the same live bacteria that you might find in probiotic pills or powders.

It's the ones that belong to these two particular 'families', or genera, that are among the first to colonise the digestive tract in humans from the very earliest days of our lives. Up front are the *Bifidobacteria*, followed later by probably the best known of all: the friendly flora *Lactobacillus acidophilus*. The name 'lacto' comes about because members of this particular family of *Lactobacilli* can make antibacterial lactic acid, which is able to ferment the natural sugars in dairy products and change them into lactic acid – hence lactic acid bacteria. (By the way, *Bacillus* means 'rod', which is the shape of this particular bacteria, and *bacilli* is simply the plural.) Although this important process was originally discovered by a scientist using milk, most of the lactic acid that's now used in food processing comes from vegetable sources such as potato, maize (corn) and molasses. That's why even vegan products can contain lactic acid and lactic acid bacteria without crossing any dietary boundaries.

Who's who?

Varying levels of different kinds of bacteria live all over our bodies: on our skin, in the urinary tract, in the vagina and in our digestive systems. The vast majority, however, reside in the intestines. That's not only important for the health of our digestive system but it's also vital for our immune system, the greater part of which lives and works from the gut wall.

So that we keep away from the complicated science of intestinal bacteria, let's – for the sake of simplicity – say that they're divided into three camps:

1 The bacteria (or microflora) in our bodies come under a general heading called commensal. It's a word usually taken to mean eating at the same table (commensal comes from the Latin: *com* – together; *mensa* – a table), but it also indicates living together in close association, which is just what we do with our own personal gut bugs. They live inside the body or on the skin and, under normal circumstances, don't usually cause disease. They could be considered as neutral, going about their work helping us to function, not bothering us directly nor harming us. If you like, think of them as your entourage. Where you go, they go. In return for their company, we provide a warm, protective environment, rich with food.

2 Some of these commensals are particularly useful and come under the heading of our good gut bugs (see opposite).

3 And then there are a few other bacteria that, given the right circumstances, can become potentially harmful or 'bad'. For example, the 'superbug' bacterium, *Clostridium difficile* or the ulcer infector *Helicobacter pylori* may live harmlessly within us but can be the cause of serious illness if the gut environment gets out of balance and allows them to multiply. *Escherichia coli* (*E. coli*) or *Klebsiella* can be cooperative in small amounts, but certain strains can be devastating to our health if they get out of control. Likewise, *Streptococcus pyogenes* survives innocuously in a healthy throat but, once it runs amok, it can cause tonsillitis, scarlet fever and, of course, that very sore and unwelcome condition known as 'strep' throat.

Did you know?
The incredibly complicated ecosystem of different bacteria that inhabit your insides isn't there when you're born. When you first arrive in the world, it's all as clean as a whistle – not a gut bug in sight.

All the colonising starts to happen immediately during and after birth, and it's this 'setting up procedure' that determines the make-up of our resident bacteria. In Chapter 22 I'll be looking at how important friendly bacteria are for mums and babies.

What are good gut bugs?

Good gut bugs are beneficial bacteria. We also sometimes refer to them as friendly flora. They improve the balance of your intestinal soup by getting the better of polluting and potentially dangerous bacteria, depriving them of food and inhibiting their growth – or, you might say, crowding them out. All these microscopic bacteria have different 'personalities' and influence our health and well-being in different ways.

They include:

Resident bacteria, the permanent inhabitants that live inside us. If you like, think of them as the home guard.
And
Transient bacteria, which are more like a visiting workforce – perhaps supply workers or travelling salesmen who are passing through. They replenish the stores and support the resident troops. We pick up transient bacteria mostly from our food supply. They may stay awhile in small colonies and give a helping hand around the place to some of the resident bacteria. In fact, they get on well with the locals who are generally pleased to see them, because the new arrivals produce by-products that the residents need in order to keep the digestion working and the intestines healthy. But once their work is done, they don't hang around; in fact, they actually die (sob!) and then get flushed out of the gut with other wastes.

When it comes to the different types of bacteria in probiotic supplements, most are destined to be transient, although a few will actually 'book a room' and move in with the existing inhabitants for a while, so becoming temporary residents themselves. But, whichever is the case, none of these friendly flora have long lives, which is why it's important to provide the body with probiotics on a regular basis.

What are bad bugs?

Bad bugs are harmful or pathogenic[JB] bacteria, the kind that spit toxins and can cause intestinal putrefaction (bad smells and decay). Remember: a pathogen[JB] is a prime mover of disease, capable of causing poor digestion, digestive ulcers, bloating, diarrhoea, constipation and gut infections. In the worst-case scenario, an overgrowth of certain types of bacteria has also been implicated in much more serious illnesses such as pneumonia, inflammatory bowel disease, pancreatitis, degenerative brain disease and multiple organ failure.

Jargon buster

Pathogens are any opportunists (especially bacteria, but could also be worms [helminths], protozoa, a virus like HIV or a fungus such as the yeast *Candida albicans*) that cause disease. A pathogen can't create disease all by itself, but if the conditions are right, it will multiply and that's when it becomes a troublemaker. Think of them as hostile agents. **Pathogenic** means something that causes disease or is capable of doing so. The words 'pathogen' and 'pathogenic' come from the Greek words *pathos*, which means disease, and *genesis* (no, not a pop group; it means bringing something into being, in this case, illness).

What do good gut bugs actually do?

Opposite are just a few of the tasks carried out by our multi-talented microflora. They're involved in:

1 **Keeping the system moving**. They're in charge of an odd-sounding but very important action called peristalsis[JB]: the movement of food and wastes through the intestinal tubing. Friendly flora also improve bowel movements and reduce the risk of bowel disorders, easing the symptoms of irritable bowel syndrome, diverticular disease and constipation, which, itself, is a known risk factor for colon cancer.

> ## Jargon buster
>
> **Peristalsis** is the term used to describe the muscular squeezing that helps to push food – and later on, waste products – along the length of the intestines. If good gut bugs are in short supply, the 'pushability' of this rubbery tube is affected, food sticks around for too long and can go very badly off! Probiotics do a great job of keeping everything moving.

2 **Reducing the risk of infection**. Another really important job good gut bugs have is priming (preparing and training) the immune system. Our good gut bugs are involved in the workings of all kinds of cells that protect us against disease. Not only can they decrease the duration of colds and respiratory infections; they're also capable of controlling and limiting the growth of unwanted and unfriendly opportunistic 'guests', including bad bacteria, yeasts (candida) and parasites. Caring for our internal environment is one of the tasks they most enjoy. By marshalling all their friendly like-minded pals to guard areas of the gut where harmful pathogens and toxins would otherwise hang about, they push the bad bugs out of their comfort zone. Not unlike moving intimidating thugs away from street corners.

3 **Taking care of the mucous membranes**. Beneficial bacteria look after something we call mucosal integrity; in other words, strengthening that important mucous-membrane defence barrier that makes up the lining of the gut; they also stimulate the production of mucins, the proteins in mucus that lubricate and protect our 'inside' skin, and secrete nutrients, which are used for tissue repair.

4 Protecting the system against SIBO (small intestinal bacterial overgrowth). They use clever tactics to undermine the activities of troublesome bacteria in the small intestine (that's where most of your digestion takes place). SIBO is one of the things being investigated as a possible trigger for irritable bowel syndrome (there's more info for IBS sufferers on page 213).

5 Looking after digestion and absorption. Because good gut bugs aid the digestion of our food and absorption of nutrients, they have a big say in how well nourished we are. They increase the absorption of minerals and are responsible for making B vitamins (which in turn are needed by the nervous system, and the skin, hair and nails; for eye health, energy production and other essentials, including helping us to burn calories) and also for production of Vitamin K_2, which is important for blood clotting. They also make special nutrients known as fatty acids, which are essential for a whole host of different processes. Good gut bugs are great at relieving digestive disturbance such as bloating and wind. One of their particular talents is the ability to digest lactose (see below).

6 Knowing their enzymes. Beneficial bacteria work to prevent the breakdown of certain not-so-desirable enzymes in the body, ones that might otherwise cause trouble by contributing to the production of cancer-causing agents. And good gut bugs are in charge of manufacturing an obliging enzyme known as lactase, which encourages the digestion of lactose – the sugar in milk which, because it's often not digested properly, can cause much discomfort for many people.

7 Dealing with diarrhoea. Good gut bugs can make a big difference to the duration and severity of diarrhoea, whether it's the result of antibiotics or is caused by bacterial infection. They can lessen the risk of real horrors such as *Campylobacter*, reduce the side effects caused by treatment of the superbug *Clostridium difficile*, cut the chances of infective or travellers' diarrhoea by helping to prevent food poisoning and protect against rotavirus (a common cause of severe diarrhoea in young children).

8 Cooling down inflammation. There are many studies showing that our good gut bugs have anti-inflammatory abilities. This is exciting because inflammation is known to be a major problem in a long list of diseases, including immune disorders, allergies, infection and fever, and could also be a factor in heart disease.

9 Helping to protect us against urinary tract and vaginal infections. They're really smart when it comes to improving the balance of friendly flora in and around your urogenital bits and pieces, so there's less risk of the body being affected by bladder or vaginal infections, discharge, thrush or the more serious condition of candidiasis.

The future for probiotics

'There is no doubt that the large and varied collection of microorganisms associated with the human body has a profound influence upon the health and disease of the host (that's you and me) ... Whilst much of the science and the products involved have concentrated on the intestines, we shouldn't forget that microbe populations occupy every exposed human surface. It shouldn't be surprising that, in the future, probiotics will be used to treat ailments other than those related to the gastrointestinal tract.'

Jeremy Burton PhD, personal email to the author, 20 July 2009

How do they get out of balance in the first place?

Believe me, it's easy. Let's start with a good example: notch up a not-so-great diet and some skipped and snatched meals here and there; make sure there's a thoroughly inadequate intake of fruits, vegetables and dietary fibre and too much refined and processed food; then throw in a few other negatives, such as stress, overwork, too little sleep, a bit too much alcohol, a few hormonal fluctuations, the effects of cigarette smoke (passive or direct) and the un-avoidable effects of living in a modern polluted environment; top it all off with a patch of not-so-good health, a gastric upset, maybe surgery or chemotherapy, or the use of different medicines, especially antibiotics, anti-ulcer drugs, steroids, or spermicides and, hey presto, it's no wonder that the intestines – where most of your good bacteria reside – don't function as they should. Not only that, it's also been shown that there are sometimes other hidden enemies such as antibiotic residues in meat, poultry and dairy foods, and in river and drinking-water supplies. Once the critical balance of good bacteria is compromised, the bad bacteria waste no time in grabbing any opportunity to take over.

Did you know?
You're absolutely full of bacteria.
Bacteria are usually only seen through a microscope (many of them resemble stumpy little sausage or egg shapes). Depending on the conditions within the body, some bacteria are considered good and helpful, some are neutral and others are putrefactive, causing rot and corruption, and encouraging disease.

A huge population

We all cohabit with trillions of these teeming little creatures. Estimates of as many as 90 to 100 trillion have been bandied about – an extraordinary number almost beyond comprehension. What's really staggering is the fact that, even though figures vary slightly between different experts, it's generally agreed that there are ten times more bacteria in the gut than the total number of cells in the whole body. Or put another way, there are more bacteria in just one human digestive system than there are people who have ever lived on the planet earth up to this point in time! This colossal quantity is generally believed to be made up of between 400 and 500 different types of both helpful and unhelpful micro bugs, although more recent investigation suggests that the number could be much higher. In case you find it easier to relate to weight rather than to numbers, you may like to know (or perhaps you'd rather not) that, at any one time, you're lugging around anything between 1 and 2 kilos of bacteria (roughly 2–4lb), just in your intestines!

If hazardous ones take hold, they can rapidly reproduce and, in the process, produce toxic chemicals that can cause serious damage to tissues and cells within the body.

One good example of this is the *Streptococcus pyogenes* bacterium, which is responsible for 'strep' throat and tonsillitis. Another would be pathogenic *E. coli*, a name forever associated in the public's mind with food poisoning, but also the cause of other infections, too. Normal *E. coli* is well behaved and sometimes even helpful, but if there's a problem in the home (inside us) and perhaps a lack of parental control, it can cross that fine line into an underworld of delinquency and criminal behaviour.

The idea behind using probiotics as supplements is that they join forces with the body's naturally occurring battalion of beneficial bacteria so that, together, they can make the best possible defence against potentially harmful nasties.

Snippet
The complex combination of bacteria that inhabits your body is so individual that it could be as unique as your DNA or your fingerprint. So, although certain species of microflora are common among lots of people, the make-up of your own personal population will be exclusive to you.

Viruses, yeasts and parasites – and the clear-up squad

Apart from the regular riff-raff of the not-so-friendly contingent in your intestines, there will also be other ugly customers, including viruses, yeasts and parasites. If you're reasonably healthy, you'll also be host to plenty of law-abiding bugs getting on with jobs such as manufacturing vitamins, breaking down dietary fibre and generally keeping the ugly customers to a minimum. Another part of the team is the uniformed branch of hard-working probiotic police who patrol the alleyways and clear out undesirables who lurk about causing general mayhem in the bends and crevices.

Probiotics are mostly bacteria, although there are other helpful substances known as probiotic yeasts that also come under this heading.

Getting the balance right

It's actually quite difficult to get any perspective on the kinds of numbers involved in total body bacteria and, to be honest, you don't really need to. What's important to understand is that having the right balance of healthy bacteria in the gut is vital to our survival. Symptom profiles suggest that many people could be suffering from bad bug overgrowth that could be very easily corrected by consuming regular probiotic foods and/or supplements, all helped along by an upgraded diet (see page 42). In practice, I certainly see huge improvements in many patients when probiotics are supplemented.

How many good gut bugs should you have?

Do an Internet search and you'll be faced with something in the order of 2.5 million options for sites claiming that the ideal numbers should be 85 per cent friendly flora versus 15 per cent unfriendly, but that most of us have the opposite; in other words, 85 per cent undesirable and only 15 per cent of the happy lot. This ratio has been quoted and repeated so often that it would be easy to accept it as established fact. Except that it's not.

These figures could never have been anything more than a rough guess; unfortunately, a wrong rough guess. There are so many bacteria – many still unidentified – that it simply isn't possible to come up with a precise quantity. This is confirmed by a report from the FAO, which tells us that up to 70 per cent of the gut microflora commonly categorised is 'new to science'. UK-based probiotics expert Dr Nigel Plummer agrees that the 85:15 ratio is nonsense. He suggests that, in the large intestine, the ideal share is 50:50; that's 50 per cent bifidobacteria (good guys) to 50 per cent bacteroides (not so good!) and that the only people likely to meet this half-and-half target are vegetarians. Those on high-meat diets don't come close; in fact, they're more likely to have 95 per cent bacteroides – the bad stuff.

All we can really say at the moment is that when the gut is healthy, and when normal balance is maintained, the good bacteria will keep the nuisances under control. And balance seems to be the key word here. The ideal circumstances are those where the beneficial bacteria predominate over the potentially harmful types.

But what about those bad guys?

Don't panic. Even in an ideal situation there will always be bad bacteria around. That's how it's meant to be. The danger arises if the number of good gut bugs is allowed to dwindle too far. When that happens, the system gets swamped with toxins, cellular debris, chemicals, pus and bile – ideal conditions for the not-so-friendly, and smelly, toxin-producing bad guys to behave like the thugs and vandals they really are. And believe me, there's nothing they like better than to have a regular and thoroughly disgusting binge, slurping on all that debris. Once gorged and bloated, they get on with their favourite business of multiplying like mad and taking over. Inevitably, this damages the environment around them. That's what vandals do. They can also upset the immune system and trigger inflammation. In the process, they disrupt your digestive system, increase the risk of infection and encourage all kinds of illnesses.

The good news

There are three easy ways to keep harmful and undesirable bacteria firmly under control:

1 Do whatever you can to create the right environment in your intestines so that it's the perfect place for good gut bugs to thrive.

2 Eat a diet rich in prebiotics: foods that give special support to your gut flora (see page 68).
3 Make sure that the gut receives a regular supply of good-quality probiotics.

How do we do that? Let's find out.

2.

Get Yourself a Good Gut Upgrade

‘Live in rooms full of light / Avoid heavy food / Be moderate in the drinking of wine / Take massage, baths, exercise, and gymnastics / Fight insomnia with gentle rocking or the sound of running water / Change surroundings and take long journeys / Strictly avoid frightening ideas / Indulge in cheerful conversation and amusements / Listen to music. ’

Aulus (or Aurelius) Cornelius Celsus (circa 25 BC – circa AD 50). Roman historian. His encyclopaedia *De Medicina* is considered one of the finest medical classics

The idea behind the Good Gut Upgrade is to give you some help right away. Use this chapter as a starting point and, as you progress through the rest of the book, keep coming back here to remind yourself to introduce one or two new changes every day.

You might wonder how some of the recommendations below can have anything to do with your gut flora, but every suggestion is included for good reason. First of all it's important to remember that around three-quarters of all your immune system (the internal army that protects you from disease) is created in – and works out of – the intestines and that your body's defence force can suffer if your digestion is poor, or if your digestive system is malfunctioning. It's also easy to forget that absolutely everything – every cell, every organ, every body system – is interconnected in some way and that the majority of functions are interdependent. When things go wrong, there can be a negative knock-on effect right down the line. Although your gut flora support you, they also need support from you. And this is where the Good Gut Upgrade comes in.

With the amount of essential tasks at work and at home that most of us have to get through each day, it's no wonder everyone seems overworked or exhausted. You may have reached the stage where you think your body is nothing more than a machine, programmed robotically just to make it through from breakfast to bedtime. The last thing you can spare is time to be ill.

Because probiotics provide such vital support to our immune systems, I'm convinced that they can actually save us precious time, by helping to keep us well. Of the many tasks they're responsible for, reducing the risk of infection and keeping the digestive system working properly have to be two of the most important in terms of time saving for us. The benefits are even greater if probiotics are used as part of a protective package, along with a few important dietary and lifestyle changes.

Why you need an efficient digestive system

Unlike repairing a malfunctioning engine, when the human digestive system goes belly-up there's much more to getting it better than simply replacing this or repairing that. When your intestines aren't working as they should, there's going to be a pretty strong chance that you won't digest your food as well as you might, which means that you probably won't be absorbing the nutrients you need to keep yourself in the best shape, nor will you be eliminating efficiently, allowing wastes to build up and toxins to flood back into the bloodstream.

By ignoring the importance of good digestion, you leave yourself open to lowered immunity and a greater risk of being run-down or under par. When digestion is dodgy and the immune system is struggling, you also hugely increase the risk of a whole range of minor and major health problems, many of which we'll be talking about later.

There's no doubt that without proper nourishment over the long term, all body systems may eventually suffer to a greater or lesser extent, even if you don't notice any symptoms at the outset. In particular, your resistance to infection and ill health won't be so strong. The Good Gut Upgrade is designed to give your digestive system that all-important lift.

Can diet really be so important?

Look at it this way. Would you ever consider spending £100 on groceries and then coming home and throwing half of it straight in the bin? No, of course not. But it's highly likely that you're doing just that without even knowing it. If your system isn't working as it should – and especially if you're having to deal with any of the conditions that we talk about in Part Two – it's possible that you're not digesting or absorbing the nourishment you need to stay healthy in the long term. I guess you could say that half your shopping bill is going down the toilet!

Don't leave it until it's too late!

One of the most distressing parts of my job is seeing patients who are referred by the doctor because they have all kinds of health problems that are being caused or aggravated by addiction to entirely the wrong foods. Worse still is hearing someone tell me that they'd rather put up with their pain, their indigestion, their excess weight, their diabetes, their high blood pressure, elevated cholesterol or risk of heart attack, than improve their eating habits.

Listen. Healthy eating really isn't difficult. Yes, there are some things you might have to cut down on if you're going to make a difference to your health – and to your good gut bugs – but nutritious food, carefully chosen and properly prepared, is no more difficult to achieve than trying to decide which pizza to buy or which takeaway to order.

I feel so strongly about this and have seen such wonderful results in people who have taken on important dietary changes that I make no apologies for groaning on about it.

Here's what to do to make the difference

First, chew your food more thoroughly.

You may think this is trivial, but it's not. Who do you know who doesn't gulp their food? We all do it every now and then but an awful lot of people eat too quickly at every meal. What they don't perhaps realise is the devastating effect that such haste could be having on their long-term health. Great granny was right: chewing everything 30 times or more really is good for you.

The advice I usually give to patients is to 'drink your solids'. In other words, don't swallow solid food until it is pulped by teeth and saliva to a semi-liquid. It should be chewed until it 'disappears' down the throat without much assistance. This action not only adds valuable digestive enzymes from saliva (especially helpful if you're eating something starchy or sweet) but also means that food is broken down more efficiently, taking the strain off the stomach and reducing the risk of digestive discomfort.

The rest of your gut will be really grateful for this extra effort, too. By using the teeth to smash food, and especially to break up the dietary fibre into tinier pieces, you give proper support to your intestines and your gut flora. Failing to chew food properly leads to more than inadequate digestion: it can encourage overgrowth of bad bacteria and all the problems that go with it (see Chapter 10 on dysbiosis). And it could also affect the body's protective army: your immune system. If your immune system isn't in good shape, then neither are you. Taking time over each mouthful also encourages you to relax – again, all the better for helping absorption.

How can you put the brakes on?

One good tip to help you slow down is to get into the habit of resting your knife and fork or spoon on the plate between mouthfuls. Chew one mouthful thoroughly before you load up with the next one. If you watch other people eat, mostly you will see them doing exactly the opposite: operating a kind of speed-eating system so that almost nothing is chewed properly at all. Some people tell me that they do this because they're really hungry, but it's worth knowing that the appetite will be far better satisfied if you chew properly and eat slowly.

And here's something else to think about: it takes an enormous amount of energy not only to digest our food but also to absorb the nutrients from it and then get rid of the waste, so anything you can do to take the strain off the digestive system will be welcome. If your body isn't coping well with this important job, it means it's having to work a lot harder than if you gave it a bit more support. And we don't just need that body fuel to sustain our physical energy. It's also vital for topping up the nutrients we need to stay healthy.

Eating out?

Don't gallop from starter to main course to dessert. I know some people say they feel honour bound to eat all the courses because they were included in the price or because they don't want to upset the cook, or they can't avoid overeating because the person who does the cooking makes the portions too big. Come on – is that the best excuse you can come up with?

Overloading the stomach is of no help at all to the intestines. One or two courses should adequately satisfy the appetite. Chat, chill, read a magazine, look out of the window, pace yourself.

Whether you're eating out or at home, try to introduce the same rules for yourself as people in the Mediterranean countries who take their time over their meals. And remember this: when you've finished you should have space left for another few mouthfuls; in other words, feel comfortable – not bloated or suffering indigestion.

Eat regularly

It makes much better health sense to eat regularly than going for long periods without food. Some people think that avoiding breakfast or not bothering with lunch and then eating only in the evening will reduce their total calorie intake and help them to lose weight. In fact, the opposite is true. Running on empty all day and relying on supper to get you by can, for some people, actually result in an increase in weight problems. It certainly does absolutely nothing for your blood sugar levels, nor does it help your intestines to function at optimum level. Even the most nourishing of foods can't be broken down properly if you overwork the digestion by eating too much at one sitting. Smaller, more frequent meals are far more likely to be digested efficiently and the calories from them burned off before bedtime. If that's not possible, at least try to have access to healthy snacks throughout the day and take five or ten minutes to sit down and enjoy them.

Never, ever, under any circumstances, eat on the move

And definitely don't eat at your computer, your desk or while you're driving. Make every effort to get away from work situations, and sit at the dining table, or relax outside – in the garden or just on a chair outside the back door, or find a bench in the park. Sit down for your meals and snacks, and stay seated for a minimum of ten minutes after you've finished eating. Give yourself time to unwind. A relaxed stomach will digest far more efficiently than a tense one.

Breathe more deeply

Most people don't breathe deeply enough. Yes, sure, but what does this have to do with digestion? Improving the way you breathe can have a range of health benefits. Chinese philosophy has it that anxiety, worry and stress affect the lungs, which in turn can lead to a dysfunctional large intestine. Improving the quality of the breathing is said to increase the energy flow between these two organs. In my clinic, I've seen so many improvements in people who've introduced simple, daily deep-breathing exercises into their routine that I now explain the techniques to almost every new patient. So why not begin right now: first, take a slow, deep breath right into your belly and let it out in a big sigh. Then do it again. This is one of the best remedies for releasing tension.

Check your posture

When the chest muscles become cramped and tight, it's easy to mistake the discomfort for digestive or heart problems. Leaning forwards or sitting in a slouched position is something many of us do without realising it, often as a result of ageing, back pain, intense concentration or simply bad body positioning. Abdominal cramps, heartburn and hiatus hernia may be relieved by improved posture.

If you suffer with persistent back pain or have repeated periods of chronic indigestion and tests can find nothing wrong, consider seeing a chiropractor or osteopath for a course of treatment. Poor posture as well as spinal lesions can alter the nerve and blood supply to the gut, affecting the way your food is digested.

Loosen your belt and your waistband

Tights, girdles, belts, skin-hugging jeans, restricting panties, tight bras, or loads of Lycra that stop you breathing out properly – all these things make it more difficult for your digestive system to work efficiently.

Get moving

Like it or not, regular exercise is as important as healthy eating. Apart from the obvious benefit of burning calories, physical activity is also a vital factor in maintaining a balanced bodyweight and improving circulation. Weight-bearing exercises like walking, cycling, sports and gym workouts are, of course, essential for healthy bones, but they also reduce the risk of heart disease and stroke, and they improve the way the body copes with the stresses and anxieties of everyday living. Exercise is vital to improving gut function and is believed to lower the risk of serious bowel disorders by as much as 40 per cent!

If you're struggling with a health problem or disability that prevents you from walking regularly or taking other more vigorous exercise, the simplest and easiest movements – deep breathing, massage, arm stretches and shoulder rolls – can still make a beneficial difference.

Get those bowels working

Once a day is regarded by most people as healthy, but you might be very surprised to know that large numbers of people go to the toilet three times a week or less. This is really dangerous because constipation is one of the biggest risk factors for colon cancer. If you're someone with a really sluggish bowel or you have a partner, friend or member of the family who suffers, I urge you (and them) to read Chapter 16 on constipation.

Make every possible effort to avoid cigarette smoke

Cigarettes do your intestines no favours at all; nor your lungs, obviously. Neither is it good for your sense of taste, your body odour, your breath, your dental bills, or your premature wrinkles.

What's more, the damaging effects of sidestream smoke on non-smokers is so well known that nothing excuses smoking in the house or the car when there are non-smokers, especially young children, around.

In case you didn't know this, cigarettes not only have a hugely detrimental effect on the digestive system and on the bowels but they also cause the stomach to overproduce acid and are implicated in ulcers. Apart from the known links to lung cancer and heart disease, it seems that cigarettes can also increase the risk of far more serious gut disorders such as Crohn's disease and ulcerative colitis. Nicotine addiction, dependence and withdrawal are now extremely well understood and there are many ways to help yourself quit.

I often see patients who are seriously ill just because they smoke. They look terrible and often feel terrible and yet, believe it or not, many of them make no attempt to give up. Some have even admitted that they like it so much they would rather die young! If you're a smoker, I make no apology for including this example of how smoking shortens your life:

Every cigarette is estimated to reduce a smoker's life by 14 minutes. That means a smoker loses nearly 5 hours of living for every packet of 20, and for every five packs, life gets shorter by nearly a whole day. If that wasn't enough, it's been estimated that smokers wrinkle 5 times faster than non-smokers! What they don't realise is that all the time this is going on, they're wrinkling on the inside too.

Be diet wise

Increase your intake of vegetables and salad foods. Even if you're not all that keen on these kinds of foods, there are lots of ways of eating more of them without really noticing. There are plenty of tips throughout the book.

Eat more fresh fruit, but do so on an empty stomach; in other words, between meals or as an entrée before other food. Fruit should be a priority in any healthy diet but, for some people – especially those with a dodgy digestive system – mixing fruit with other foods seems to affect not only the way that fruit is assimilated in the stomach and the small intestine but also can be a common cause of bloating, gas and acid indigestion. Instead of enjoying that fruit salad at the end of the meal or the apple you were going to have after you've finished your sandwiches, do it the other way round. We eat melon as a starter, so why not eat the fruit salad or the apple before the meal?

No one really knows why this works, but my experience with patients suggests that it's definitely worth a try. Fresh fruit and unsweetened or freshly squeezed fruit juices also make good snacks between meals (instead of coffee and cake or biscuits), and they add nicely to that all-important five-a-day quota. Drink fruit juices and fruit smoothies before or between meals, too. Also, anybody with any kind of digestive or bowel upset may find that it helps to avoid starchy pastry with acid fruit, such as an apple tart, plum crumble or strawberry sponge. It's interesting that people often blame the fruit for their griping gut pain when the problem is actually caused by the unwise combination.

Not too hot – nor too cold

It's worth considering that stomachs were invented before cookers and refrigerators. Very cold or very hot (hot temperature and hot spicy) foods can disturb digestion and absorption. Very hot spicy foods can also have a detrimental effect on the pancreas, a complex and hard-working gland that is responsible for producing enzymes to help you digest your food, and hormones to keep your blood sugar balanced.

Be honest with yourself about your alcohol intake

It's easy to drink more than we realise, especially when we're eating out. Make a conscious note of how much you have, and if it's regularly more than the recommended maximum of two units of alcohol per day, do your health a favour and cut down. Find out what a unit actually looks like (see overleaf). Drinking a glass of non-carbonated mineral water before a meal can help to dampen the desire for alcohol and also reduces the tendency to overeat.

> ### What is a unit?
> One unit is equivalent to 8g or 10ml of alcohol, which is about what you get in a single 25ml measure of spirits, half a pint of beer or one very small glass of wine. A unit will also depend on how strong your drink is; for example, half a pint of regular lager is 1 unit, but the same quantity of some continental lagers could rate 2 or 3 units. A whole pint of strong beer or cider contains 3 units. One small glass of wine can count as 1 unit but wine varies tremendously in strength, and most people don't use small glasses, certainly not wine bars or restaurants. It's the same with spirits when some pubs serve 35ml measures. So it's easy to be fooled into drinking more than you realise.
>
> Check out these websites. They have easy interactive ways of checking your intake:
> www.drinkaware.co.uk
> www.units.nhs.uk
> www.drinkingandyou.com

Don't eat wheat

We're all encouraged to believe that wholegrain wheat is a good way to increase our intake of dietary fibre, but high-fibre wheat may not suit us all that well. Too much of it can impede weight loss and cause discomfort and bloating, and more and more people are finding themselves sensitive to wheat and related products. Wheat bran may still be recommended by some doctors and dieticians as a useful dietary fibre but, in my experience and that of many of my colleagues, it can be devastatingly harsh to a tender intestine. Personally, I would have it banned along with margarine and politicians. Even in a mixed-grain cereal, for example, you very often find that wheat is shown as the first ingredient, which means it's predominant.

There are much better options available. For more information, see page 53.

Eat more fabulous fibre

Instead of relying on wheat for your main source of dietary fibre, try oats, brown rice or rye-based foods, which are all supportive of your good gut bugs. So are brown basmati rice, Ryvita crispbread, whole rice crackers or rice cakes, rice pasta, rice macaroni, porridge, oat muesli, rye bread or the less well-known grains such as kamut, quinoa or buckwheat. They all make great and very healthy alternatives to the troublesome wheat that you find in so many cereals and in bread, biscuits, pastry and cakes.

Spelt, or espelta, is a type of wheat that, unless you've been diagnosed as seriously and properly allergic to all kinds of wheat, is usually better tolerated and doesn't seem to aggravate bloating or other digestive discomfort. It may take a bit of sleuthing in specialist markets, delicatessens or health-food stores but the effort is really worth it. And I'm certain that your good gut bugs will be much happier about it. Many supermarkets also now cater for people who prefer to avoid wheat.

Don't forget that, even with all these deliciously different grains, it's a mistake to rely totally on cereals for our roughage. We need other kinds of fibre too, in particular from fruit and vegetables. That's another reason why it is really worth aiming for that minimum five-a-day target.

Push up your daily fibre quota

1 Cook potatoes in their skins, eat wholegrain pasta and brown rice instead of white pasta and white rice.

2 Avoid refined cereals such as cornflakes, slimmers' cereals, anything that crackles when you push your ear to the bowl or that's loaded with a sugar or chocolate coating, and products that claim to sustain you but leave you feeling empty half an hour after breakfast. Check pack labels. Most cereal brands are heavily loaded with sugar (often 20 per cent or more), even the so-called healthy ones. Whole oats and wheat-free muesli are far better options.

3 Include chopped Brazil nuts, unblanched almonds or chopped walnuts (unless of course you have a nut allergy), sunflower and pumpkin seeds, dried apricots, prunes, dried

---

figs and sultanas. Add them to breakfasts or baking, or just snack on them.

4 Try these ideas: eat fresh fruit between meals, add a fresh juice as a starter to a meal every day, introduce vegetable soup to your menu and add a side salad to your main meal. If you do, you'll be well on your way to a healthy intake of dietary fibre and achieve that essential fruit-and-veg target all at the same time.

5 Use the lists on pages 103 and 104 to remind yourself which are the best choices.

Never axe flax

One of the best favours you could do for your body is to add flaxseed to your daily routine and regard it as a regular food. Flax (also called linseed) contains what is known as a mucilaginous fibre – a word that describes perfectly its soft, gentle and kind action on the gut. Combined with water, it becomes jellylike or slithery and is just the right type of fibre to keep those bowels working. And your good gut bugs positively love it!

There's important information on flax in Chapter 6. Please read before you buy.

Cut back on cow's milk

Did you know that two-thirds of the world's population can't digest milk and never have been able to? That's because of evolution. Where there were no cows, there was no cow's milk and so the digestive systems of those peoples evolved without a requirement for milk-digesting enzymes. Where there were cows, milk wasn't processed or pasteurised and still contained natural enzymes that helped its digestion. When pasteurised milk or milk powder has been introduced into the diets of people who are not used to it, the result is often abdominal pain, bloating, nausea and disturbed bowel function – all the symptoms of lactose intolerance.

Good gut bacteria play a role here because they help us to digest lactose, the natural sugar we find in milk. This is useful if you like to drink milk but have been suffering from bloating and gas.

However, even with the help of probiotics, I don't recommend drinking it by the glass or pouring it on to cereal. Cow's milk is often touted as a rich source of calcium, and it's true that this certainly applies if you are a calf. But whether or not it's just as beneficial for humans is a much-argued point.

Many of us are simply 'maldigesters' of milk products, and my experience in practice definitely suggests that, in most cases, people feel better when they don't drink cow's milk. There seems no doubt that it's mucus-forming and can still play havoc with the digestion even if the milk sugar is properly broken down. If you suffer from sinus problems, repeated ear infections, runny nose, asthma, eczema, stomach acidity or irritable bowel syndrome it can really be worth giving up the white stuff to see if symptoms improve. Of course, unless you are sensitive to this food, a small amount in tea is usually no problem.

What are the milk alternatives?

Unsweetened soya milk doesn't work well if you pour it straight into coffee, because it curdles. But it's fine if you mix it half and half with water, heat the liquid in a pan and then pour it onto the coffee. I don't think it's very tasty in tea so, if cow's milk is a problem, the only answer is to get used to weaker black tea or go green or herbal with lemon. It's good to do because putting milk into any kind of tea tends to wipe out its medicinal properties. Good-quality green tea is healthily antioxidant. For cereals, you might use soya milk, oat or rice milk, or add yoghurt instead. Goat's or sheep's milk, and yoghurts made from them, are widely available. As to worrying where you'll get your calcium, there is no need to be concerned. This mineral is ubiquitous in our diets, being available from so many foods, that it's almost impossible to avoid it unless for some reason your diet is very restricted. Yoghurt, cheese, canned sardines, fortified soya milk, almonds, sesame seeds, sunflower seeds, tofu, oats and pulses (peas, beans and lentils) are all sources of calcium. Lots of vegetables also contain worthwhile amounts of this important mineral.

Drink more water

Most of us don't drink enough water, but there's a very good reason why we should. Apart from the fact that low water intake can aggravate many health problems, the body simply doesn't function properly without a regular supply of water throughout the day. For starters, it's a fact that dehydrated brains don't function. Which is why, when you're dry, you make more typos on the keyboard, find it harder to add up or remember names, lose concentration and feel really tired. Lack of water is said to be the number one cause of daytime fatigue. Good gut bugs are more likely to thrive when you give them the right kind of dietary fibre and the fluid it needs to move properly through the intestines.

Here are some easy ways to increase your fluid intake:

1 First, take the glass and the cup or mug you use most of the time and, with a measuring jug, find out how much each one holds.

2 Next, buy yourself two 1-litre bottles of mineral water or, if you prefer, one 2-litre bottle (the point is to make sure you know what 2 litres actually looks like). Refill these each day from a filter jug or larger container and use them as your daily reserve. If possible, use glass bottles. (Plastic contaminants – also called endocrine disrupters – can affect the water that is stored in plastic bottles. It's already known that, once in water supplies, they're capable of changing the sex of fish!)

3 Every time you have a glass of water or juice, a mug of soup or a cup of tea, write down the quantity. Keep the list going for three days. At the end of day three, add up the total. If it's less than 6 litres (10½ pints) altogether, you might need to increase the amount of water you are drinking. Or add a couple of cups of herbal tea. Or make sure that you have a bowl of soup or an extra glass of fruit juice. Remember that a probiotic drink will also count towards your daily fluid intake.

4 Always have a glass and some filtered or bottled water ready for use in your bathroom. Every time you go to the toilet, whether that's to empty your bladder or your bowels or just to wash your hands, have a drink of water. The same applies at work – let water out, take water in.

5 Put a glass of water beside the bed and if you don't drink it during the night, then drink it as soon as you sit up ready to get out of bed in the morning.

6 And always try to carry small bottles of water in the car, in your bag or on your bike. But don't be tempted to drink water that has

been previously frozen in plastic bottles or where plastic bottles have been left in the sun. There are concerns that the chemicals given off under those circumstances may cause serious health problems. Glass may be heavier but healthier.

7 Have water with you when you go walking. There are plenty of portable containers that fix on to straps or belts.

8 Don't let your body fool you into believing that just because you're not thirsty, you don't need to drink. As we get older, the mechanism in the brain that's supposed to send us the important message to take fluid on board gets rusty and forgets to pass the message down the line. So you need to take charge and make sure that you remind yourself to drink.

9 It's worth bearing in mind that although regular tea, herbal tea, juices, soups and probiotic drinks count towards your daily intake, coffee and alcohol do not. Sorry about that. So watch your intake of these two. It's fine to drink one or two cups of coffee per day or a glass of wine, but you can't count coffee or alcohol in your fluid quota because they are dehydrating. Coffee (especially if it's strong), canned and bottled soft drinks containing caffeine, and all kinds of alcohol are sworn enemies of the digestive system, especially the liver and the pancreas – and the body has to work a lot harder to process them.

Eat plenty of probiotic and prebiotic foods

Include probiotic and prebiotic foods in your diet – you'll find a list on page 85.

Steer clear of grumpy-gut foods

There are some foods that I would class as cantankerous and disruptive as far as the smooth running of your body is concerned. They seem hell-bent on upsetting your digestion or they refuse to be digested properly at all, or they aggravate blood sugar and cholesterol levels. Or, they delight in pushing up your weight and increasing your risk of heart disease and diabetes, or perhaps loading unwanted chemicals into your liver or binding up your intestines and making you constipated. These are the foods that also do no favours for your gut flora.

As you'll find out later on in *Good Gut Bugs*, the type of food we eat determines how much (or how little) support and assistance we give to the beneficial bacteria that work so hard to keep us healthy. That's why it's important to avoid things like fry-ups, pizzas, burgers, red meat (especially pork), packaged ready meals, sugar and sugary foods, cakes, biscuits and desserts, which are high in fat or sugar and not kind to the intestines. It's also best to steer clear of anything containing artificial additives, sweeteners, colours, flavours, stabilisers, emulsifiers and preservatives. It's also why the list of swaps that follows is such an important guide to upgrading your diet. Your good gut bugs will definitely thank you for it.

Swaps

This list of swaps is a simple system designed to:

1 Increase the quality and variety of your food choices.
2 Increase the nutritional value of your diet.
3 Reduce your intake of unhealthy fats.
4 Balance your bodyweight.
5 Encourage you to include the kinds of foods that nurture your intestines so that they function as efficiently as possible.
6 Give your gut flora the best possible chance of keeping you healthy.

The column on the left contains foods that many of us would choose or use without thinking. The column on the right has the healthier options. Follow as many of the recommendations as you can, introducing a few at a time over the next few weeks.

Instead of this	Go for this
Processed cooking oils Note: Most mass-produced polyunsaturated oils (sunflower, corn etc) are heat-treated, stripped of nutrients and processed using chemical solvents. I'd recommend you avoid them.	For cooking, cold-pressed extra virgin olive oil is best but don't let it smoke! Olive oil is great for dressings or for drizzling onto cooked vegetables, jacket potato or salads. Or add to soups or pasta just before serving.

	Try cold-pressed nut or seeds oils, such as flax, pumpkin seed, safflower, sesame, sunflower, walnut, avocado or grapeseed oils – add a couple of teaspoons into juices or smoothies. Important: • Store all cold-pressed nut and seed oils in the refrigerator. • Never let any kind of oil get so hot that it 'smokes'. This damages the oil and isn't good for you.
Polyunsaturated margarine-type spreads or low-fat spreads Note: Many spreads are processed using chemical solvents and contain hydrogenated vegetable oils. I definitely don't recommend them, whatever kinds of promises they may make about what they can do for your health.	A little non-salted butter or olive oil. If you store olive oil in the fridge, after a few days it thickens and becomes 'spreadable'. Or use ripe avocado pear or hummus as alternative savoury spreads.
Salted snacks such as crisps and peanuts Note: If you can't live without the occasional pack of crisps, buy the better quality brands. Avoid those that contain additives or hydrogenated vegetable oil and search out brands that are cooked in olive oil.	Almonds, Brazil nuts, hazelnuts, macadamia nuts, pecan nuts, walnuts, sunflower seeds and pumpkin seeds. Not only plenty of nutrients, good dietary fibre and healthy oils but also lots of prebiotic potential too! Note: Obviously you won't include nuts if you are allergic to them!
Chips/fries	Scrubbed, sliced potatoes sautéed in a little extra virgin olive oil make a tasty alternative and will also have a much lower fat content as a result.
Deep-fried food	Choose alternatives that are stir-fried, steamed, grilled or oven-baked.
Sweets and cakes	An occasional dessert or cake should be enjoyed but you already know that it's not a good idea every day. A fresh juice, smoothie or a piece of fresh fruit can be just as delicious, far more nutritious and kinder to the waistline!

Instead of this	Go for this
Sprinkling sugar and artificial sweeteners onto foods Note: Sugar puts a huge strain on the body, using up loads of body energy and wasting heaps of valuable nutrients. It overworks the pancreas and increases the risk of type-2 diabetes. It's not good for the digestion either, feeding any yeasts that are in the gut and causing bloating and weight gain.	It's really worth trying to wean yourself away from both these sweetenings. If you have an incurable sweet tooth, change to natural cane sugar and then ease up by a few grains each day. Alternatively, use a small amount of best-quality honey. Fructo-oligosaccharides (FOS) (see Chapter 4) can be bought as a sprinkling sugar. It's good for the gut and suitable for diabetics too.
Puddings/desserts/ice cream Note: As a treat, home-made ice cream is a better option than factory-processed alternatives.	Soaked dried fruit compote is delicious. Or for a nourishing dessert, mash a banana with half a carton of sheep's or goat's milk yoghurt and a teaspoon of honey. Chopped fresh figs, stewed with ginger, honey and red wine, and served with Greek yoghurt, make a very healthy pudding, rich enough to satisfy the sweetest tooth.
Chocolate	The only cure for chocoholism is willpower! Enjoy it on special days, but aim to cut down. When you do eat it, choose real dark chocolate, which, in small amounts, is actually good for you. Keep it in the fridge and eat a couple of squares at a time.
Fruit juices that come in bottles or brick-pack cartons Note: Watch out. Processed and UHT juices are not recommended here. Many of them are heat treated, reconstituted and contain colourings, hidden sugar and acids. This applies particularly to some kinds of 'fresh' orange juice, which may not be as 'real' as you think.	Fresh juices from the chill counter, especially grape, apple, pomegranate and pineapple. Top tip: Consider investing in a juicing machine, smoothie maker or an ordinary food blender to create your own smoothies at home. Use the type that leaves the pulp in the drink, otherwise you're throwing away valuable dietary fibre and lots of nutrients. Two pieces of fruit can make a substantial drink. Try blending an apple with a kiwi or nectarine with banana, or a small bunch of grapes with a ripe pear. Wash and peel and remove any stones or seeds before blending.

Coffee, tea and cola Note: There's nothing wrong with a cup of quality black tea or coffee, but don't overdo it. However: • An excess of coffee can overwork the adrenal glands, liver and pancreas, and increase the effects of stress. • Black tea contains valuable nutrients, but too much can affect the body's absorption of iron. • Too much cola could result in less calcium and magnesium being taken up by the body.	If you enjoy the occasional cola, choose the regular kind and avoid 'diet' or 'zero' versions that contain artificial sweeteners. Herbal teas? Not everyone likes them, but they really are worth investigating; for example, best-quality green tea is a rich source of antioxidants. Don't make herbal tea too strong. Serve with a slice of fresh lime and, if you need it sweeter, half a teaspoon of honey. Fresh juices diluted with 50% water are refreshing and can make a substantial contribution to your daily intake of fluids.
Pork and beef	These two meats are rarely well digested, and less so as we age. They can also increase the levels of uric acid in the system. Fresh fish, especially oily fish, poultry or occasional lean lamb are better alternatives.
Breakfast cereals that contain wheat or corn (both common allergens) Note: Always check the labels. Nearly all supermarket-packaged cereals are very high in sugar, even those that are supposed to be healthy high fibre.	Oat porridge, oat muesli, gluten-free muesli, rice puffs or millet flakes. Your health-food store or delicatessen (and, in some European countries, the pharmacy) is usually the place for non-wheat cereals. Or make your own muesli. Mix a couple of tablespoons of fine oat flakes with chopped walnuts, Brazil nuts, almonds, dried apricots, dates, a sprinkling of sunflower seeds and some sultanas. Serve with plain yoghurt, oat milk, rice milk or unsweetened soya milk.
Cow's milk	Unless you are sensitive to this food, a small amount in tea should be no problem. However, I don't recommend drinking it by the glass or pouring it on to cereal. Try unsweetened soya milk, oat or rice milk, or yoghurt on cereals. Goat's or sheep's milk, and yoghurts made from them, are widely available in most supermarkets.

Instead of this	Go for this
Cow's milk cheeses Note: The calcium from cow's milk cheese is more bio-available to the body than that from the milk itself, so in moderation this can be a nutritious food. But it can also be mucus forming, so use only occasionally. Avoid sliced, smoked and processed cheeses.	The problem with cheese is that we all tend to eat too much of it. Cutting down on quantity is often all that's needed. However, if cow's milk cheese doesn't suit you, it's worth knowing that nearly all major food stores have at least two different varieties of sheep's and goat's milk cheeses that are just as nutritious and can be easier to digest.
Smoked foods, including kippers, smoked salmon, smoked meats	Occasionally is fine, but not regularly. Smoked foods contain nitrates (so do hotdogs), which have been linked to a host of health problems including a greater risk of juvenile-onset diabetes, leukaemia and potential damage to the developing foetus.
Ordinary mass-produced bread Note: Most mass-produced bread is high in salt.	Bread wheat is a common source of bloating, digestive discomfort and apparent weight gain. Many people are wheat-sensitive. If you are one of them, rice cakes, Original Ryvita, oatcakes or oat biscuits might suit you better.
Pasta Note: Pasta is often blamed for being a high-calorie, weight-increasing food. But it's more likely that the cheese content of the dish is responsible. Try the pastas opposite with a vegetable/tomato topping instead.	People who have a sensitivity to bread don't always have difficulty digesting pasta. However, if you love pasta, but are sensitive to it, spelt or kamut pasta, rice macaroni or quinoa spaghetti are delicious alternatives. Available from health-food stores and some delicatessens and supermarkets.
Battery eggs Note: Just Google the words 'Life of a battery hen', read some of the results and then see if you think that creatures who suffer such cramped conditions and appalling stress can really produce healthy eggs.	Free-range eggs are better; organic free-range are better still. People who have been diagnosed with high cholesterol are sometimes told to avoid eggs, but this is based on old thinking. Eggs can make an important contribution to a healthy diet because they contain significant amounts of protein and vitamins B_2, B_{12} and D, as well as the mineral iodine. Unless you have an allergy to eggs, there is no need to avoid them. Boiled, poached or scrambled are best. If you're going to fry them, the tiniest drop of extra virgin olive oil is enough.

Canned vegetables Note: Always check the labels. Many canned foods are high in salt or sugar, or both.	Fresh and frozen vegetables. Blending home-cooked vegetables into a purée is a great (and 'invisible') way to add extra nourishment to soups, stews and sauces.
Salt, ketchup, mayonnaise Note: Use organic ketchup, make your own mayonnaise and try sea salt instead of ordinary table salt.	First of all, be honest with yourself about the quantity you really use; it could be more than you realise. When you're searching the supermarket shelves, remember that sea salt, organic ketchup and mayonnaise made with olive oil make better choices – but don't overdo them. Dressings made with extra virgin olive oil or walnut oil and balsamic vinegar are a healthy option for salads.
Low-fat foods including low-fat yoghurts, spreads, mayonnaise and anything labelled 'diet', 'reduced fat' or 'fat-free' Note: Steer clear of any that contain artificial colourings or flavourings, modified starch, artificial sweeteners, stabilisers or emulsifiers, which is also likely to include most of those labelled 'low-fat' or 'zero fat'. Remember that manufacturers often use chemical solvents to extract fat from certain foods.	Use the real, unadulterated alternatives. Don't rely on food producers to cut your fat intake at source on your behalf. The best way to reduce fat in your diet is to monitor it yourself by avoiding high-fat foods, and processed and hydrogenated fats.
Pre-packaged convenience meals Note: These are almost always very high in salt and often contain plenty of additives.	Prepare meals from your own fresh basic ingredients so that you know what goes into them. They don't need to be elaborate or take long to prepare. Simple meals are often the best.
Eating out	If you eat out regularly, avoid fried foods, rich dishes and sauces. Say *no* to potatoes, *resist* the bread. Instead, always ask for extra vegetables or salad.
Stuck in a rut? Always choosing the same old stuff? Did you know that the vast majority of our meals are based on only a handful of foods, in particular wheat and dairy?	Introduce more variety. It's the easiest way to get more nourishment into your diet. Be more adventurous with your menus. Buy a wider selection of fresh fruits and vegetables. Promise yourself you'll try a new fresh food each week, something you've never eaten or cooked before.

3.

Where Do They All Hang Out?

It has been observed that one's nose (the extreme outpost of the face) is never so happy as when thrust into the affairs of others, from which some physiologists have drawn the inference that the nose is devoid of the sense of smell.

Ambrose Bierce, *The Devil's Dictionary*

In Chapter 1 I mentioned the almost unbelievable number of microscopic creatures that live inside us. If there are so many bacteria, how is it that there's enough room for them and us? Where do they all live?

There are lots lurking around your armpits, in your groin, under your nails, on your hands, in between your toes and, not surprisingly, on your perineum, the area between the anus and the genitalia. And there are plenty crawling all over your arms, legs, torso, face and scalp, too. But they're not just *on* us, they are, of course, *in* us as well.

Come with me on a journey through the digestive system and take a look for yourself. Knowing a little about the major bacterial battlegrounds in our bodies can help us to see why friendly flora are so important to so many different areas of our health.

? Did you know?
The reason why our 'inside skin' is constructed so differently from our 'outside skin' is because the gut wall has to be permeable to allow nutrients from our food supply to be able to move through it.

Think of the gastrointestinal tract as a kind of extended ring doughnut. If you picture the doughnut hole as the space within the gut wall, you can see that it is, in fact, part of the outside world even though it's really inside the body. Once we grasp the idea of this 'hollowness', it makes it easier to understand that food isn't truly inside the body until it's been absorbed through the gut wall. And, as you'll see later, the bacteria in our bodies play a really important part in this process.

Your gut

First of all, let's sneak inside that slimy old inner tube that doctors call your gut or gastrointestinal tract, which runs from the mouth and oral cavity, down the oesophagus (gullet), into the stomach, on to the small intestine, and then into the large intestine before arriving at the rectum and, finally, that ring of muscle known across the land as your anus.

The gastrointestinal tract isn't just a lifeless bit of piping connecting one part of the body with another. It's a vital transport link that distributes nutrients to different locations via a complicated and very clever food-processing workshop (your intestines). You shovel food in at one end and the body ingeniously processes all the constituents, taking what it needs to run the system and pushing the unwanted wastes out of the hole at the bottom. Even more importantly, it's an incredibly intricate ecosystem that supports the trillions of microorganisms that live in or on the gut wall and in the gut contents, especially the colon.

When it doesn't work smoothly

Sometimes, though, the usual coordination gets fouled up and doesn't work as well as expected. Foods are not always digested properly. This may be simple, as in lactose intolerance, where undigested milk sugar from the small intestine passes to the colon, allowing bacteria to use it for a gas-and-bloating party. Or it may be more complicated, as in leaky gut syndrome, candidiasis or food allergies. Suffice to say that substances which wouldn't normally be allowed anywhere near the bloodstream manage to sneak through the gut wall and create all kinds of havoc with the immune system. Instead of being ejected, waste products get to hang around, allowing bad bacteria to multiply and toxins to be reabsorbed. One way to help avoid these problems is to make sure that the gut is well cared for (Chapter 2, page 35 will tell you how to do this) and that the body receives a regular supply of probiotics (see pages 244–5 and 273).

Let's take a closer look at the bacteria in your mouth

Now here's a nice, warm, moist place that all kinds of bacteria absolutely love – around 600 different types, in fact. Many of them are well behaved, but there are others who are real troublemakers, wreaking considerable havoc on their environment. The result is usually a build-up of complex bacterial communities that combine into plaque and can lead to bleeding gums, tooth decay and periodontal disease. Accumulation of undesirable bacteria can also occur in places such as the tongue. This is not the smooth surface that people think it is, but more of a damp and pitted carpet where bacteria compete to take up residence and make lots of nasty smells resulting, for us, in bad breath.

If the diet is right and the environment of the mouth is healthy, helpful bacteria will support us in the battle to keep the gums, tongue and teeth in good condition. But create the wrong environment and bad bugs will grab any excuse to go where they don't belong. If we already have a build-up of bacteria within the mouth, especially if we have a weakened immunity, this can allow some of the normally friendly bacteria to cause infection, disease and abscesses. Chronic oral problems such as periodontal disease, which have strong associations with bacterial infection, are also implicated in heart and circulatory disorders, preterm labour and diabetes.

I'll be looking at mouth freshness and oral health in more detail – and what you can do to help yours – in Chapter 12. You'll also get a glimpse of the likely havoc that could be taking place in your mouth as a result of bad bug overgrowth.

Down into your breathing apparatus

Bacteria are bound to congregate in the upper reaches of this tube, known as the respiratory tract, simply because it's so conveniently close to your mouth and therefore adjacent to where the food is delivered. Apart from those that munch on food waste, there are also the microscopic bugs you collect with every in-breath. Each time you do this, air passes through the nose or mouth, then through the voice box, down the windpipe, and into those two breathing bags we call the lungs.

Any bacteria that manage to avoid getting caught up in the hairs inside your nose will probably attach themselves to the membranes in your throat and your pharynx[JB]. Large communities of bacteria exist harmlessly in the area of the nasopharynx; although, in children, this site can also be a reservoir for the kinds of bacteria that cause ear infections such as otitis media or painful infection of the Eustachian tubes (the tubes to the ears). In adults, viral and bacterial infections that take hold in the upper respiratory tract can be responsible for painful afflictions such as sinusitis. Mouth breathers have less protection from airborne bugs because more bacteria will manage to make it at least as far as the windpipe or trachea[JB]. The good news is that certain types of what we now consider 'good bacteria' can help to protect against such infections.

Jargon buster

The **pharynx** is the section that begins at the back of the throat behind the nose and ends at the junction between the top of the trachea or windpipe and the oesophagus (the tube that goes from your mouth to your stomach). If the pharynx gets infected, the result is pharyngitis (not to be confused with laryngitis). Although it may sound similar, the pharynx is entirely different to the larynx, which is your voice box.

The windpipe (**trachea**) is the airway that extends from the larynx down into the lungs.

Down to your lungs

The lower part of the respiratory tract, which includes the trachea and the lungs, generally doesn't get colonised with many bacteria unless the lungs become infected. This is because any bugs that make it past the nose or mucous membranes usually get pushed out and upwards by tiny little hairs, called the cilia, which protect the windpipe.

All the while, your friendly bacteria are working hard to discourage any bad bugs that could cause mouth and throat infections. They do this by attaching themselves to the surfaces of the membranes inside the mouth and throat. Once in place, they not only help to produce natural antibiotic substances but they also inhibit the trespassers by restricting the food supply they need to multiply. But if conditions are hostile (the mouth is too acidic or the cells are lacking in oxygen), instead of the good bugs crowding out the undesirables, the reverse happens and unwanted bacteria get to do their favourite thing: reproduce and run riot.

What's happening in your gullet?

The swallowing tube that carries food from your mouth to your stomach is known as the gullet or oesophagus and it's located just behind the windpipe and the voice box. The openings to the gullet and the voice box are very close together in the throat. Usually, food is kept away from the windpipe by a flap of skin called the epiglottis, which closes over when we swallow, thereby protecting the voice box and the trachea, and stopping us from choking. Well, that's what's supposed to happen. Unfortunately, sometimes it isn't as effective as it should be, especially if we try to swallow without chewing properly, if we laugh, cough, sneeze or breathe in suddenly while we are in the process of swallowing or if we talk at the same time as chewing.

This is no place for bacteria. A few may manage to cling on temporarily, but with the constant swoosh of food and fluids that rush by at various intervals on their way to the stomach, it's not an easy area in which to get a grip.

Now we've arrived in the stomach

The stomach is a part of the body that's entirely taken for granted, often overfilled and regularly abused. Apart from acting as a temporary storage container for all our meals, it churns our food around, mixing it with gastric juices and reducing it to a semi-liquid called chyme. This amazing food bag is also a waystation, which holds the mashed-up food so that it isn't dumped too quickly into the next port of call along the line: the small intestine.

As far as bacteria are concerned, because it's such a very acidic place, you'll never find huge numbers here. The few good gut bugs that do decide to make their home in the stomach (this includes some strains of *Lactobacillus*) need to be what are known as acid-tolerant. They're up against hydrochloric acid (known as HCl), which is so strong it can dissolve iron filings and would burn holes in your stomach lining if it wasn't cushioned by a special protective layer. This is good for us, because HCl is one of the first major lines of defence against anything dangerous that you might inadvertently swallow, such as a food-borne bug.

In most cases, bad bugs can't put up with acidic environments; that is, unless the stomach is, for some reason, swamped with a really large dose of pathogenic bacteria, such as in a food that has degenerated so much it has gone off and therefore become hazardous.

For more info
An overgrowth of *Helicobacter pylori* bacteria is known to be responsible for causing nearly all ulcers. It's a problem that's far more common than you might imagine, and it's possible to be a carrier without having any obvious symptoms. *H. pylori* manages to sidestep stomach acid by moving away from the acidic areas and hiding in among the protective mucus and skin cells that line the stomach wall. (See Chapter 20 for more.)

Most bacteria live in your intestines

Sometimes called the small bowel, the small intestine, is an amazingly complex 6.4m (21ft) of sausage-like tubing that weaves its way from the exit in the lower part of the stomach to something known as the ileocaecal valve, which joins the small to the large intestine. This junction is on the lower right side of your abdomen (if you're looking down), just to the inside left of where your right hipbone juts out.

The small intestine has three sections and it's in this truly amazing length of miracle conduit that most of our digestion and absorption takes place. Some bacteria inhabit this long and busy road but, because parts of it are acidic and other areas are busy with bile or digestive enzymes, it's not such a comfortable stopover for large quantities of good gut bugs. The further we progress down this internal tubing, we find that the acidity gets less and, as a result, the numbers of bacteria increase.

The duodenum

The first 30cm (12in) after the stomach is called the duodenum where the majority of the minerals from our food are taken across into the bloodstream. In a healthy body, you won't find too many bacteria in the duodenum, because the upper section will be receiving semi-liquid from the stomach, which, of course, is very acidic. That means the environment as far as microflora are concerned will still be hostile. However, our acid-tolerant *Lactobacillus* family of friendly flora do hang out in this space, albeit temporarily, along with some *Streptococci*, plus small numbers of *Escherichia coli* (that's *E. coli*) and yeasts.

Snippet
The wall of the small intestine is a little like a kind of capillary mat with lots of tiny protruding fingers and millions of perforations all aimed at absorbing essential nutrients from the gut into the body. Only things that are allowed into the bloodstream can normally pass through. But where the

ecology of the intestines is disturbed and inflammation runs riot, the little holes can become much bigger, increasing the risk of all kinds of unwanted debris escaping into otherwise secure areas.

The jejunum

Next comes the jejunum – which deals with water-soluble vitamins, carbohydrates (also called starches) and proteins. As we progress through the different sections of the small intestine 'going south', there is less acidity and lower levels of oxygen, conditions that encourage microflora to multiply.

The ileum

The microflora carry on multiplying when they get to the last part of the small intestine, called the ileum. This piece of piping is in charge of fats, fat-soluble vitamins, cholesterol and bile salts. Here we find more natural inhabitants such as *Lactobacillus acidophilus* and *Bifidobacteria* doing daily battle with unwanted pathogens (bacteria, protozoa, parasites and yeasts). In any gut on any day of the week you might find small numbers of *Candida albicans* (a natural inhabitant yeast that can also sometimes get out of control), likewise the bacteria known as *Clostridium difficile*, so common in hospital environments, *Klebsiella*, found in patients with pneumonia, *Salmonella* and *E. coli*, both associated with food poisoning, *Cryptosporidium* (a water-borne parasite that can cause a devastating diarrhoeal illness called cryptosporidiosis) or *Giardia lamblia*, a very resistant parasite believed to be rampant in care homes and day centres, responsible for gas, watery stools, diarrhoea and, in severe cases, malnutrition. What stops all these predators running amok are your beneficial bacteria. But if the balance between the supportive and the destructive has been disrupted in any of these areas, expect chaos.

When support breaks down, bad bugs take over

When bad bugs take hold, they steal nourishment from your body, feeding off your internal food supply and lazing around while they wait for undigested food particles to decompose – because that's just how they like them. When they run riot like this, it can lead to a condition known as small intestine bacterial overgrowth or SIBO (see Chapter 18).

If the mucosal lining of the gut isn't properly protected by beneficial bacteria, it's likely to become irritated and inflamed, allowing bacteria, yeasts and unwanted components to work their way into the bloodstream. When this happens, so many alarms go off at once that it causes absolute mayhem in the immune system, which lurches into a kind of manic overdrive. This increases the likelihood of allergies and hinders the absorption of nutrients. Inflammation and malabsorption very often result in leaky gut syndrome (LGS). There are also particular problems in conditions such as coeliac disease and inflammatory bowel diseases like Crohn's or ulcerative colitis.

> ### Did you know?
> Dietary fibre – of the right kind – plays a really important part in the survival of good gut bugs in the large intestine. It's here that fibre is broken down, water is reabsorbed, and wastes are prepared for elimination. Just for this job alone, the body needs around 1.4 litres (2½ pints) each day to do this. Since most people don't seem to drink anything like this amount of fluid, this might be one of the reasons why so many suffer from constipation. Probiotics can also help in stimulating the muscular movement of the intestines as well as the transit of wastes. I'll be looking at the importance of dietary fibre in Chapter 6, and at how probiotics can help bowel problems in Part Two.

The biggest and busiest contingent of body bacteria settle in your large intestine

Also known as the large bowel or colon, the large intestine is much shorter in length than the small intestine – around 1.5m (5ft). (It's called 'large' not because of its length but because of its chunky diameter.) There are five distinct sections and hundreds of thousands of bacteria living here.

The first part, the ascending or proximal colon, leads off from the ileocaecal valve down by your right hip bone. From there, it travels in a more or less straight line upwards to the right side of your waist.

Then it turns across your middle (to the left if you're looking down at it and to the right if you're looking at someone else's) to the opposite side where it turns again, this time down the left side of the body.

Not surprisingly, this section is called the descending, or distal, colon. At this point it sort of 'disappears' towards your back into the final segment, the sigmoid colon (so-named because it's supposed to be shaped like the eighteenth letter of the Greek alphabet, Σ, although it's really more like the letter S), and, at last, arriving at its ultimate destination, the rectum and the anus, the end of the journey.

By the time all the residues of digested food have finished travelling through the small intestine and arrive in the large one, most of what's left is a load of mushy fibrous fluid. It's up to the large intestine to sponge the excess water from these leftovers which, by now, are looking increasingly like sludgy poo.

In amongst it all, there are also likely to be a fair old whack of bacteria, maybe some parasites, and without doubt the residues of any medicines you've taken along with the remains of ingested chemicals, artificial food additives and other toxins discarded by the liver. Not stuff that you really want to hang on to.

Keep moving

Here's a major reason why it's such an important thing to keep up our intake of friendly flora, make sure that we eat the right type of fibre and take enough fluid: because they all function together to give these wastes the best chance of passing through at the right speed. If they move too quickly, water isn't reabsorbed and stools are very loose or liquid; too slowly and the bad bacteria get to party in the mud – the wastes putrefy, dry up and stick to the colon wall, narrowing the tube and blocking the walls.

Ideally, there should be plenty of good bugs in this last section of tubing. In a healthy body, it's a probiotic paradise – and a busy one at that. Here, you'd find helpful flora, such as *Bifidobacteria*, encouraging the absorption of certain nutrients from your food, assisting in the manufacture of essential vitamins, and knocking the living daylights out of those undesirables such as pathogenic *E. coli.*, *Shigella* (a common cause of diarrhoea in children), another food-poisoning favourite, *Campylobacter*, or perhaps the potentially plague-like *Clostridia*, to name but a few.

Internal deodorant

Probiotics work hard here to keep the place smelling sweet, just as they do in other parts of the body. Well, reasonably sweet. All poo has a natural odour, and everybody prefers their own to someone else's – but bump off the good bugs and you'll notice the seriously bad smells rising up to greet you straightaway! It's easy to tell if they're getting out of control. Just take a sniff. When there's been an ecological disaster – such as when the whole lot has been annihilated by taking antibiotics – it's no wonder that noxious gas and smelly stools can be two of the side effects.

Unfortunately, it's a bacterial fact of life that bad bugs smell … um … bad.

A good example of how good gut bugs can make the difference is what you find in a baby's nappy. The odour that rises from the stools of a bottle-fed baby is particularly strong and not at all pleasant, because the levels of friendly bacteria are generally quite low. In contrast, the smell from the soiled nappy of a breast-fed baby isn't at all off-putting. That's because it's rich in *Bifidobacteria*.

Snippet
Just as bad breath might indicate bad bacteria in the mouth (and also the stomach), a strong stink from anywhere in or on the body nearly always indicates an overgrowth of undesirable bugs. If you notice any not-so-nice pongs about your person, or anyone else's, such as foulness of the feet, groin or underarms – or embarrassingly smelly farts – you can bet your bippy that bad bacteria will be at the bottom of it.

More from the lower half of the body

Let's pay a quick visit to the urogenital bits and pieces while we're wandering around down here.

Under normal healthy circumstances, there shouldn't be any bacteria to worry about in your kidneys or in the ureters (the two tubes that feed urine to the bladder). This situation could change if you succumb to a kidney infection. But there are a couple of other warm, moist places that act as a heavenly haven for several different kinds of bugs or yeasts. In the urethra (the peeing pipe between the bladder and the outside world), there could be *Staphylococcus epidermidis*, *E. coli* or *Proteus mirabilis*. And in the vagina, you might find the inevitable yeasts but also *Staphylococcus*, *Streptococcus* and *Corynebacterium*.

Now come with me and find out about some seriously special foods that are essential for supporting the good bacteria in our intestines.

4.

Prebiotics – Your Probiotic Support Group

> ‘Illnesses hover constantly above us, their seed blown by the winds, but they do not set in the terrain unless the terrain is ready to receive them. ’
>
> Claude Bernard, French physiologist

Notice that in the title I said *pre*biotics. I know we've been talking throughout the book about *pro*biotics and how helpful they can be towards achieving better health, but it's important to realise that they're not self-supporting. They only get to do their best work if *we* help *them*. This doesn't only apply to the probiotics we take as supplements or foods but also to the resident friendly flora that we first talked about. We need to create the right environment within the body so that all our friendly flora have the best chance of doing their job, and we do this by eating foods called *prebiotics*.

Think of it like this. You have a piece of land where you're trying to raise a crop. Imagine that the soil is terrible. Without any help at all, there's a possibility that something might grow but it probably won't be very good. You might try throwing fertiliser onto the ground and this could improve things but, if the field is rubbish to start with – perhaps it's stony, full of debris and choked by weeds – the crop will never reach its full potential. An already weakened crop might fail entirely and be overrun by pests or diseases simply because the tilth was never prepared properly or the nutrient levels weren't right.

Inside your body is similar, so swallowing supplements in isolation is never going to be enough. To ensure the best circumstances for good gut bugs to thrive and work efficiently, it's vital to prepare the ground first – what 19th-century scientists Louis Pasteur and Claude Bernard referred to as 'the terrain'. This means making sure that we supply the body with the right kinds of foods. That's because probiotics and prebiotics are synergistic to each other. Combining the two creates a kind of teamwork. By making sure that we nourish our bodies with both *pro-* and *prebiotics*, the resulting benefit is likely to be far greater than by using one or the other in isolation.

Ideal partners

Some press reports have inferred that prebiotics are somehow a better option than probiotics and that probiotics are not as helpful as we once believed. This is nonsense. If good bacteria are in short supply, prebiotics will simply turn their attention to the bad guys and feed them instead! Until, that is, more good guys come along and take preference. So it's perhaps worth pointing out that it's not a choice between either increasing probiotics or eating more prebiotics. One is not better than the other. We need both. We need friendly, helpful probiotic bacteria and we need the prebiotic foods to feed them.

Just to clarify:

*Pro*biotics are the friendly flora.
*Pre*biotics are the food substances that support them.
*Pre*biotics are *not* bugs, bacteria or any kind of living organism.

Important new findings

The big interest in prebiotics isn't just some kind of fad that's here today and gone tomorrow. The excitement is ongoing because of the recognition that what happens in our intestines has major consequences for our health. Specifically, researchers are investigating how prebiotic substances may have the ability to stop pathogens (the bad guys) sticking to the gut wall, how they work in balancing blood sugar and cholesterol, help us to control our weight, speed up the transit of wastes, ease the symptoms of inflammatory bowel disease and, hopefully, have a significant effect in lowering the alarming rates of colon cancer.

Feeding our friendly flora

The important thing to know about the prebiotic parts of any particular food – and the reason why they work so well – is that they don't get digested. In fact, they positively resist it. That's how it's meant to be. When we eat foods that have a prebiotic component, the small intestine will extract any useful nutrients on the way down and then give the undigested bits a free pass to the next department, in this case the colon or large intestine. But they're not wasted. In fact, they serve as welcome grub for our good gut bugs, who grab hold of it, chomp it up (actually, they ferment it) and use it, among other things, to help produce more friendly flora who then carry on the good work. So while *pro*biotics busy themselves throughout the digestive system, *pre*biotics are effective only in the large intestine.

Where do we find prebiotics?

In non-science-speak, prebiotics are simply naturally occurring components found in a whole array of delicious foods, such as wholegrains, fruits and vegetables, which work closely with the good bacteria in your gut. They're also found in live yoghurt and a long list of fermented foods (Chapter 5). Most people are aware that dietary fibre is good for us and it's interesting that many foods containing dietary fibre are also prebiotic – although it doesn't follow that every fibrous food will have prebiotic qualities. I'll explain more about this important aspect shortly.

Pages 85 and 103 have detailed lists that you can work from, including suggestions for prebiotic foods that are even suitable for people who generally gag or grimace whenever the word 'vegetable' is mentioned in their presence! Did you know it's estimated that only 8 per cent (yikes, that's fewer than one in ten!) actually get around to eating the recommended minimum of five servings a day of the green, orange, red, yellow and purple stuff?

What did you say your name was?

The word 'prebiotic' is relatively new to the English language. It was first coined in 1995 by Professor Glenn Gibson, now at the Department of Food Biosciences, University of Reading, and Dr Marcel Roberfroid of the Université Catholique de Louvain in Belgium. They defined prebiotics as 'Non-digestible food ingredients that beneficially affect the host by selectively stimulating the growth and/or activity of one or a limited number of bacteria in the colon, and thus improve host health.' This statement was updated by Dr Roberfroid in 2007 (and endorsed by the Food and Agriculture Organization of the United Nations) to describe 'a selectively fermented ingredient that allows specific changes, both in the composition and/or activity in the gastro-intestinal microflora that confers benefits upon host well-being and health'. Gibson and Roberfroid are, by the way, two of the leading researchers in this field.

Prebiotics are finding their way into functional foods

A 'functional food' is one that either already contains a proven active ingredient or is fortified with some kind of 'extra' that has been verified and confirmed by research to provide a particular health benefit. Or put another way, it's a food or drink that, in addition to its usual content, includes an ingredient that has the power to help prevent disease. Here are a few examples:

- One of the first things to become a functional food was salt when, at the turn of the 20th century, iodine was added because it was known to prevent abnormal enlargement of the thyroid gland, known as goitre. Now, of course, we tend to use too much salt and, along with it, have created new health risks, especially that of stroke and high blood pressure.

- Cranberry juice is a functional food because it's known to help lower the risk of urinary tract infection. People often think that it kills the bacteria that cause infection, but this isn't the case. It works because the active ingredients inhibit the attachment of *E. coli* to the bladder wall. In plain English, instead of hanging around and setting up a nasty little community of bad bugs, the *E. coli* finds it too uncomfortable to stay, so it moves on and gets washed away when you pee.

- Chickens who have therapeutic doses of omega-3s added to their feed produce 'functional' eggs, because omega-3s have a proven health benefit to the human heart and circulation.

- Any food that has calcium added, such as soya milk or orange juice, is considered a functional food.

- White bread on its own is hardly healthy and doesn't do much for anybody's 'function', but fortify it with fibre and you create a functional food, because dietary fibre has a host of established health benefits. It doesn't necessarily mean that the white loaf with added bran is as good as the real, unadulterated wholegrain, but it's a step in the right direction for folks who think that the brown version is only for health freaks.

Food technology to the rescue?

Now, prebiotic 'extracts' are being added to a whole range of supermarket products, disguised so cleverly that you would never know they were there. At the time of writing *Good Gut Bugs* there are no precise guidelines governing the use of the term 'prebiotic' on food products – although this will soon change. What you do see are pack flashes boasting that an item is, or contains, a prebiotic. You don't need to look very far. They're showing up in everything from bread to breakfast cereals, yoghurts to chocolate spread and snacks to supplements.

Adding 'pre-mix' prebiotics to your diet can be a useful shortcut if you're lacking in these essential foods. There's no doubt that some products are excellent, but it's not a good idea to rely on branded items as a complete answer to your daily needs. The good thing is that packaged foods sometimes tell you how much prebiotic you're getting for your hard-earned cash, but even this doesn't necessarily mean something contains useful amounts. And don't assume that simply because a product includes some supposedly healthy ingredients that the rest of it is going to be of any particular value. It may still be processed in some way or contain additives, especially high levels of sugar and salt.

These new food products aren't a licence to bunk off broccoli and sneak another burger, but it does mean that fruit-rejecting, vegetable-avoiding lovers of plastic bread or synthetic snacks might unknowingly end up being healthier than they would have been if left to their own devices. Although not everyone will agree, perhaps there's no choice but to take functional and novel foods seriously. When you consider that the current average intake of prebiotics is between 2g and 3g per day and that experts believe we need at least double this figure – and preferably treble it – if we're going to have any kind of beneficial effect on our friendly flora, these new inventions could be vital to the nation's health. If nothing else, it must be good news for those who are resolute about never changing their diets for the better.

An unbeatable team

Increasing our intake of prebiotic foods doesn't mean that we don't need probiotics. Include both probiotics and prebiotics in your diet and evidence suggests that it could be better for your health than using just one or the other. When taken together they're known as *syn*biotics, a term already being used to describe any food that has a positive pairing of both prebiotic and probiotic qualities.

A perfect example of Mother Nature's symbiosis is the cultured milk known as kefir (see page 86). Because it comes complete with its own supply of good gut bugs (probiotics) and also has prebiotic ingredients to support the production of more beneficial bacteria, it can rightly call itself a natural synbiotic.

One especially exciting piece of research was tested by the European Union-sponsored Synbiotics and Cancer Prevention in Humans Project, where a synbiotic combination of a prebiotic (oligofructose) and two probiotics (*Lactobacillus rhamnosus* GG and *Bifidobacterium lactis* Bb12) were given to patients at risk of colonic polyps (because they're considered markers for colon cancer). The results showed that there was a decrease in the uncontrolled growth of cells in the colon wall. Although only preliminary, it's incredibly encouraging to think that something so simple and so safe might have such a profound impact on reducing the incidence of this mostly avoidable disease.

What makes a prebiotic?

A lot of claims have been made regarding prebiotics that have yet to be substantiated. What's still being sorted out is which foods have the right to call themselves prebiotics and which don't. Although a great many vegetables and fruits, and plenty of different wholegrains, are known to have genuine prebiotic accomplishments, it doesn't necessarily follow that every fruit, every vegetable or every cereal is qualified to be included in the list. The same applies to dietary fibre. Just because fibre is a healthy thing to include in the diet, it's not accurate to claim that all fibrous foods are prebiotic – nor that all prebiotics come from fibrous food; for example, yoghurt, green tea and red wine (see below) could hardly be described as roughage!

So, just to recap, for a food to be classed as having prebiotic qualities:

- Some or all of its ingredients must have attributes that allow them to sneak past the normal digestive processes in the stomach or the small intestine.

- The undigested bits and pieces then need to pass to the large intestine where they get fizzed and bubbled by beneficial bacteria, otherwise known as fermentation.

- The fermentation action has to actively support the production of more beneficial bacteria.

- And finally, the whole shebang must be beneficial to the health of the host – that's you!

In the simplest possible terms, the best way to describe prebiotics is as food for our friendly flora.

How much prebiotic food should I include in my diet?

Advice about how much you need varies. Some experts recommend that we need around 5g of prebiotic each day, others suggest 7g or even 10g. A pucker Mediterranean diet, for example, has been put at anything from 12g to 18g. However, the actual figure doesn't really matter. All you need to do to make sure that you're consuming a decent quantity of quality prebiotics without any need to keep score is to:

- Include *at least* five servings a day of fruits and vegetables (and remember that five is a minimum here, not a maximum).
- Choose from as wide a variety as possible of wholegrain foods and pulses (peas, beans and lentils).
- Eat live yoghurt and/or take a yoghurt-type drink every day.
- Add a selection of other regular items from the list on page 85 and from the dietary fibre suggestions on page 103.

Good news

You might already have heard that two of life's stress-reducing essentials – good red wine and quality dark chocolate – both contain prebiotic components. But don't get carried away. Stuffing yourself with your favourite sweet treat and getting legless on the red stuff might seem like the way to prebiotic heaven, but it won't work, because it would be excessive and restrictive. To help support and stimulate all the different kinds of bacteria that live inside us, the body relies on us to feed it with a diverse selection of prebiotic foods. So unfortunately, as much as I wish I could tell you otherwise, relying exclusively on your favourite bottles of plonk and boxes of Belgians won't get you by.

A strong wind to the south?

A slight downside, particularly in the early stages of adding more prebiotics to your diet, is that you may notice an increase in – let's be upfront about it – farting or belching. I'm afraid that prebiotics have no shame! Although in the long term, this very healthy component can help to reduce bloating and gas, to begin with they may get worse. Please understand that this doesn't apply to everybody, and that the amount of gas will depend on the sensitivity and forbearance of your gut. If it's generally crabby and intolerant, gassy eruptions may be a bit more likely, but if you have a Terminator 2 intestine of steel, then you might not notice the effects! In any event, the effects are almost always temporary and are a positive sign that the prebiotics are working. A bit of bloating, a rumbly tum or a few gassy eruptions, in the short term, are surely worth it for the sake of sorting out your intestines and helping them towards functioning more efficiently.

Efficacious acacia?

A new kid on the block that's beginning to be recognised as a beneficial prebiotic is acacia bark, an extract that has been shown in studies to be especially good at encouraging the growth of very important friendly flora known as *Bifidobacteria*. Acacia may also be a worthwhile alternative prebiotic supplement for sufferers of irritable bowel syndrome.

If you decide to add a prebiotic supplement to your diet, or one has been recommended to you by your health-care practitioner and you're finding that it's giving you wind, then begin on a very low dose. In the meantime, this case history below may be helpful:

Case history

In 2008, I saw a patient who was referred with diverticulitis, constipation, high blood pressure and extremely high cholesterol. As part of his treatment, I recommended a change of diet to include less wheat bran, more oats and flax fibre, a wider range of vegetable foods, probiotic supplements and a prebiotic known as FOS (short for fructo-oligosaccharide). It looks just like sugar and is easy to take when added to cereal or yoghurt. He made good progress almost at once, but was a bit over-enthusiastic with the FOS and complained that gas was a big issue! I suggested that he cut the recommended daily amount of one teaspoon to, literally, a pinch per day for a week. Then, increase to two pinches for another week, then three and so on until he was back up to a teaspoon per day. It worked perfectly. There was no bloating and no wind problems. In less than six months, his cholesterol and blood pressure were back to normal (without drugs), he was no longer constipated, nor was he bothered by any symptoms associated with the diverticular disease.

Supplementary benefits

We've already taken a brief look at the capabilities of prebiotics, but there are other claims for their talents, too:

- One fairly immediate and beneficial effect of a high-prebiotic diet is usually that you notice more frequent bowel movements, perhaps twice a day instead of once. Constipation is the result of a sluggish colon holding up the movement of wastes; medics call it slow intestinal transit. Prebiotics support the good gut bugs and assist in pushing wastes nicely along, helped considerably by the bit of natural gas they produce during fermentation. These special foods attract water to the intestines, which swells the stool and encourages it to speed up and get the heck out of there – which, given that constipation is a big risk factor for colon cancer, can only be of benefit to you. (See Chapter 15.)

- Promising research suggests that prebiotics inhibit the formation of lesions in the gut, reducing the risk of cancers of the digestive tract.

- Like their probiotic partners, they seem to have a favourable effect on the immune system, which means that they provide additional support to the body when it's fighting infection.

- Prebiotics also chase out toxic compounds and reduce the population of harmful bacteria.
- By increasing the level of good gut bugs, some prebiotic types encourage natural antibiotic activity, which means they can hinder the growth of undesirables.
- They boost production of some really essential nutrients called short-chain fatty acids. SCFAs are what you get when prebiotics (don't forget these are the undigested bits and pieces left over at the end of the digestive process) are broken down and fermented in the large intestine. Work now being done using prebiotics is showing us that our health could be seriously compromised if we don't have enough SCFAs. Unfortunately there isn't the space available here to tell you about the very important work that they do. However, happily for us, there are lots of really appetizing prebiotic foods that can help us 'prepare the ground' in our intestines so that we continue to supply our bodies with these essential nutrients.
- Experimental studies have come up with a possible plus in the management of diabetes. In particular, FOS has been shown to lower blood glucose levels in animals. In addition, it seems to be the case that diabetics who include plenty of prebiotic foods in their diet, especially pulses and vegetables, have better control of their blood glucose levels.
- FOS also aids the absorption of the minerals calcium, iron, magnesium and zinc. However, if you use it as a supplement, remember my earlier advice: that the best benefits come with the caution 'slowly does it!'. Always begin with a pinch (literally the amount you can grab between finger and thumb) per day and work up to the daily amount recommended on the pack over a period of a couple of weeks. If you dive in at the full, recommended amount from the outset, your gut won't have time to adjust and you're likely to get temporarily gassy and bloated. This caveat also applies to probiotic supplements that contain FOS, so check labels before purchasing. FOS is great stuff for most people, but needs gentle introduction.
- There's evidence that prebiotics have value in reducing raised cholesterol and triglycerides (blood fats), thereby reducing the need to take lipid-lowering drugs.

- There's good news too when it comes to weight control. Experts in the field of gut microbiology are looking to prebiotics – as well as probiotics – as a possible way of tackling obesity.

- Prebiotics may even be able to dictate how our bodies cope with pharmaceutical medicines. Some people tolerate prescription medicines in an entirely different way from others, and researchers are pondering the possibility that our gut flora may somehow be involved. Perhaps prebiotics and probiotics might help medicines to work more efficiently? Or, perhaps, prebiotics added to drugs may also help us to deal better with the side effects?

- In practice, I've used prebiotics successfully to help lower uric acid – particularly in conjunction with supplements of probiotics and FOS (see pages 78 and 280). This can be especially helpful to people with gout and arthritis.

Later on, I'll be telling you why fibrous food is such a team player when it comes to providing the body with prebiotics and how there's so much more to dietary fibre than a daily bowl of string-and-sawdust cereal.

If you want to make a start right away, one of the easiest ways to begin creating this all-important 'terrain' is to follow the advice in Chapter 2. Otherwise, move right along to the next chapter.

5.

Gas Guzzlers: the Health Benefits of Fermented Foods

‘[We] often forget the most fundamental of all rules for the physician, that the right kind of food is the most important single factor in the promotion of health and the wrong kind of food the most important single factor in the promotion of disease. ’

Sir Robert McCarrison, 'Diseases of Faulty Nutrition', *Transactions of the Far Eastern Association of Tropical Medicine*, 1927

When we use the word 'ferment' to describe an emotion, we usually mean something that fumes or simmers under the surface. The foaming and bubbling that goes on in your large intestine isn't really all that different, although the end result is likely to be far more beneficial to your health than, say, the stress of brewing up anger.

In the previous pages, we looked at the synergistic connection between probiotics and prebiotics. The magic that makes this synergy happen is fermentation, a really important part of the workings of the human digestive system. It's something we don't often hear about but is vital to our health and survival. Scientifically speaking, fermentation is the process of obtaining energy from the breakdown of the starches and sugars that we also call carbohydrates. I suppose you could describe it as the catalyst that changes the characteristics of one thing so that it becomes something else.

An ancient tradition

Not all that long ago, before the advent of freezing, pasteurisation, industrial canning or production-line bottling, fermentation was one of only a few methods of storing food safely. Our ancestors had an innate wisdom – call it a good gut feeling – which told them that these foods were somehow beneficial. They also knew that their skins of yoghurt and crocks of fermented vegetables would stay good and fresh at the back of the cave for weeks or months. But it would be more than a few generations before Ilya Mechnikov (see overleaf), or anyone else for that matter, twigged the precise reason for their success.

Even though the alchemists of ancient Greece wrote about the chemical changes that occurred during the fermentation process, they still didn't know exactly what it was that preserved the food or provided it with such healthful qualities. The Hunzakut tribes of the Himalaya, studied so extensively by Sir Robert McCarrison, are famous for their longevity, a characteristic attributed to their simple diet, in particular its low-fat, high-fibre content, consisting of wholegrains, fresh vegetables and fruits (including goji berries and Hunza apricots), butter, a limited intake of meat and lifelong consumption of fermented milks. The Romans raved about pickled cabbage, because it tasted so good, but they had no scientific clue as to where its medicinal potential came from. How could they have known that it was the beneficial bacteria produced from the fermenting starches and sugars that acted as a natural preservative and restricted the growth of the type of bacteria that could cause food poisoning? Or that it increased the nutrient levels and made the food easier to digest? Or that it encouraged the growth of more friendly flora, which, as we've seen from previous chapters, have some amazing health-giving properties?

The role of lactic acid

The most common end product of all this fermentation activity is lactic acid, which is produced by lactic acid bacteria, such as *Lactobacillus acidophilus*, *L. brevis*, or *L. delbrueckii*. *Lactobacillus casei*, a probiotic bacteria which you sometimes see included on the labels

The Importance of Ilya Mechnikov

The first modern mastermind to switch to the idea that the type of bacteria in the intestines might have significant effects on human health was called Ilya Mechnikov. He worked out that the friendly bacteria in yoghurt had the power to crowd out pathogenic organisms in the gut and prevent overgrowth of bad bacteria.

Ilya Ilyich Mechnikov was born in the Ukraine in 1845 and died in Paris in 1916. Some translators refer to him as Elie Metchnikoff and also incorrectly as Eli Metchkinof but they're all talking about the same person. A zoologist, pathologist, bacteriologist and microbiologist, he was considered one of the founding fathers of modern immunology.

What had grabbed Ilya's interest was the fact that the rural peoples of Bulgaria seemed to live much longer than those in other countries and were generally much healthier. So he started nosing around the Bulgarian diet and found that they ate a lot of soured milks (which we call fermented dairy products), especially yoghurt. He did some tests and decided that it was the fermenting lactic acid bacteria in the milk foods they consumed that were responsible for their robust health, stronger immunity, longevity and a general lack of degenerative illness.

It was at the Pasteur Institute in Paris that Mechnikov developed his theory that the process of ageing is caused by toxic bacteria in the gut and that helpful lactic acid bacteria could therefore have the power to prolong life. He was convinced that people became sick if the bacteria in the colon were disturbed or disrupted and that by eating fermented foods rich in what we now know as probiotics, symptoms could be sorted and illness prevented. He is also believed to be the first person to use the word dysbiosis to describe a bacterial imbalance in the gut, the starting point for many unwelcome diseases.

of yoghurt and yoghurt drinks, is so-called because it comes from casein, a milk protein that is curdled by lactic acid.

Apart from yoghurt and fermented milks, lactic acid fermentation is involved in the production of sourdough bread and beer, and in preserving all kinds of vegetables, including beetroot, olives and onions. We make chutney and relishes from mixed vegetables, tomatoes, corn, cucumber and a whole array of different fruits. However, vegetables that are simply preserved in vinegar, such as pickled onions or gherkins, are not fermented and so do not contain valuable probiotic bacteria.

Asian cuisine is famous for its fermented pickles, which include cabbages, turnips, aubergines, cucumbers, tomatoes, green peppers, onions, pumpkin, butternut squash and carrots. *Kimchee* is a kind of oriental version of sauerkraut made from Chinese cabbage with added ginger, garlic and red bell pepper. The Japanese *umeboshi* is a pickled plum often prescribed as a medicinal treatment for an upset stomach.

In Africa, *magou* is a dish made from a slurry of fermented maize; cassava fruit, once it's been through the fermentation process, becomes *gari* or *fufu*. *Balao balao*, a mixture of fermented shrimps and rice is traditional in the Philippines. In the Middle East, their fermented milks are known as *laban*, and when they ferment milk and cereal together, it's called *kishk*.

Why lactic acid is so special

In all these foods, it's lactic acid bacteria that suppress the growth of undesirable bugs that would otherwise spoil the food or cause it to decompose. And it's that same lactic acid that is responsible for the sharp taste that is so familiar of fermented foods.

Lactic acid is also antibacterial – bad bugs hate anything acidic (see overleaf).

Snippet
The reason we call someone 'pickled' when they're drunk, is because of the fermentation of alcohol that's going on inside their gut.

Are we missing out?

Even though these ancient methods of fermentation are still common in many ethnic diets, they're used relatively little in the highly processed Western diet. Research proves, however, that a regular intake of prebiotic foods – and in particular, fermentable fibre – is capable of reducing the risk of a number of serious 21st-century health problems: not only type-2 diabetes, obesity, high blood pressure and elevated cholesterol but also a long list of gut and bowel disorders, including constipation, diverticulitis, haemorrhoids and inflammatory bowel diseases.

One of the most important health benefits that occurs as the result of foods being fermented in this way is that it lowers the pH (the acid balance) of the intestines. Or put another way, by making your gut slightly more acidic, the lactic acid guys create an uncomfortable environment for bad bugs who are then less likely to stick around, reproduce or cause trouble. These kinds of conditions not only help to protect the lining of the colon but, in the same way that the acid in fermented pickled foods preserves them from being spoilt by bad microbes, a slightly acidic colon deters smelly and stroppy pathogens from taking over.

There's also a big calcium bonus here. If the acidity levels are correct, it means that we're able to absorb more of this important mineral from our food. Clamber inside a healthy large intestine and you'd find that it was quite a vinegary place!

Beans means fartz?

We all know that pulse foods such as haricot beans, kidney beans, chickpeas, lentils and butter beans can make us gassy, which is why some Venezuelan scientists decided to have a go at rendering them more digestible. How did they do this? By mixing them with 'helpful' bacteria. As a result, beans can mean 'fewer fartz'. The only obvious difference is that the beans themselves taste sharper – just like other fermented foods.

Other useful organisms

Yeasts, moulds and enzymes are also part of the team that makes hops into beer, grapes into wine, flour into bread and milk into yoghurt or cheese. Inside you, a similar process is kicked off by your good gut bugs as they change the non-digestible leftovers from your diet into nourishing and useful things that you need in order to survive; in particular, essential fatty acids and further supplies of beneficial bacteria.

Active foods

Here are just a few of the foods that are said to have prebiotic activity. Notice that quite a few of them are produced using the fermentation process.

All the *Allium* family:
    Chives
    Garlic
    Leeks
    Onions
    Shallots
    Spring onions

Almonds, whole and ground
Artichokes – globe and Jerusalem
Asparagus
Bananas
Bimuno™*
Burdock root
Buttermilk
Chicory root
Cottage cheese
Dahi (home-made yoghurt)
Dandelion
Flax fibre
Fermented soya beans/bean paste:
    Doenjang
    Miso
    Tamari
    Tempeh

Ginseng
Goat's milk
Goat's milk yoghurt
Green beans
Green tea
Jícama (Mexican potato)
Kefir (fermented milk)
Kombucha (fermented tea)
Koumiss
Manuka honey
Molkosan (fermented whey**)
Oats, uncooked
Pickled vegetables:
    Gherkins
    Daikon radish
    Kimchee pickled cabbage
    Sauerkraut pickled cabbage
    Pao cai Chinese pickled cabbage
    Zha cai Chinese pickled
      mustard
Sheep's milk
Sheep's milk yoghurt
Soya beans
Tomatoes

Wholegrain breads, crispbreads and cereals

Yacón (a tuberous root vegetable related to artichoke)
Live yoghurt

*Bimuno™ is a dedicated prebiotic product (available from chemists), which can be mixed with food or into beverages.

**Molkosan Vitality (from Bioforce Dr Vogel) is a powdered prebiotic drink made from naturally lactic-acid-fermented whey. It has a positive effect on intestinal flora, contributing not only to the reduction of bad bacteria but also to the creation of an environment that supports the growth of friendly gut bugs. Molkosan also contains vitamins B_1, B_2, B_3, B_5, B_6, B_{12} and folic acid, vitamin A, beta-carotene, vitamin C, calcium, potassium, magnesium, zinc and iron. It has an excellent record in relieving intestinal complaints, including flatulence, bloating, gas and constipation.

The best of both worlds

Let's look at one particular type of fermented milk: kefir. It's interesting because not only does it provide us with a healthy whack of good gut bugs but it's also naturally prebiotic and gives genuine meaning to the words 'health food'. Studies show that it can be helpful for lowering cholesterol and blood pressure, balancing blood glucose and helping ease constipation. I've also found it a valuable food for anyone who suffers with IBS, diverticular disease, food sensitivities, and especially for candidiasis. It's a good therapeutic, too, if you've been stricken with *Giardia*, *Klebsiella* or *Helicobacter pylori*.

Kefir is believed to originate from Eastern Europe, in particular the region known as the Caucasus, and is made by combining the kefir 'grain' with milk from the sheep, goat, cow or camel. The traditional way of storing it was in skin bags, which were then hung up and swung or knocked to mix the contents. Nowadays, it's produced for wider consumption and is sold throughout Europe including countries such as Bulgaria, Poland, Russia, Latvia, Estonia, Lithuania, Ukraine, Belarus and Scandinavia – and is a regular part of the diet in all the countries that once made up the former Yugoslavia. It comes in many different guises in lots of different places; for example, you might take it straight in Spain, mix it with fruit juice in Kefalonia or sup it in soup in Denmark.

From little 'grains'

The kefir grain is not a cereal that you can grow in the ground but a combination of friendly bacteria and yeasts that are produced during fermentation. The resulting shapes look like grains and can vary in size from very tiny (like rice) to larger pieces that resemble florets of cauliflower. It's these kefir 'shapes' that are used as the starter to make more kefir, just as you would use yoghurt to make more yoghurt. Although it's traditional to use raw milk from animals, kefir will also ferment almond milk, coconut milk, rice milk and soya milk.

If you haven't tried kefir, give it a go, and if you gave up because you didn't like the taste, please try again. It's a useful and very healthy addition to any diet. Some people dislike it because it can taste quite sour (as do many other fermented foods). However, the level of sharpness depends on the type of bacteria involved and how long it was fermented. The amount of time taken to ferment can also have a bearing on the nutrient content. Highly ripened kefir may taste more tart, but the bonus of this is that, with time, the folic acid content goes up. Banana and honey (both of which are prebiotic) are especially good at disguising the sharp flavour and can transform plain kefir into a sensational smoothie.

Lactobacillus kefir is sometimes used in probiotic supplements.

Getting the benefit of probiotics and prebiotics

If you add probiotics on their own to your daily routine, it seems pretty likely that you'll see some worthwhile health improvements. Or, if you ignore the probiotics in favour of increasing the prebiotic foods in your diet, you may experience a turn for the better, or you could find that your prebiotic diet isn't helping as much as you'd hoped. If we take the research so far and add to that the weight of expert opinion, combining the two – that is, taking regular probiotics and including at least some of the foods from the lists on pages 85 and 86 – seems the very best way to go. Together they make a safe and powerful package that can be aimed not only at the relief of symptoms and the treatment of illness but also at the prevention of disease.

6.

Fabulous Fibre: How Getting it Right Could Save Your Life

‘Dear Kathryn, We are nominating you for the Nobel Poo Prize. My wife has BEEN 8 days in a row – never before happened in her life! Congrats! ’

Email to me from the husband of one of my patients. This lady, despite consuming daily wheat-bran breakfast cereal, had – until she began to follow my dietary recommendations – only ever opened her bowels twice or three times a week. On the following day, there came a brief follow-up email which read: 'Now it's 9!'

If you've read the earlier section on prebiotics, you'll already know that dietary fibre is an important part of the prebiotic team, perhaps playing a bigger part in your health than you might have imagined. Certainly, there's far more to fibre than breakfast bran as the lady above discovered to her benefit. That's why, in this chapter, I'll be looking at the need-to-know detail and giving you the low-down on the best sources. Why is this so important? Well, don't forget that many of the foods that contain dietary fibre are also prebiotic, which means that they're fully paid-up members of your probiotic support group.

Because of our fondness for highly processed foods, and the fact that lots of us aren't even close to eating the recommended daily intake of vegetables, fruits and wholegrains, experts estimate that many people, especially in affluent countries, may be consuming only a quarter – or sometimes even less – of the fibre they actually need to maintain good health. That can be extremely dangerous.

Given the near epidemic of so many potentially preventable

diseases, it should come as no surprise that lack of fibre in the diet is known to increase the risk not only of constipation, haemorrhoids and anal fissures but also of cardiovascular disease, diabetes, obesity and a range of bowel and digestive disorders including Crohn's disease, ulcerative colitis, diverticulitis and the growing epidemic of colon cancer.

What is fibre?

Dietary fibre – we used to call it roughage – acts rather like a broom that helps to push faeces along the length of the large intestine, preventing a build-up of solids and keeping the contents of the bowel moving and the walls of the tube free and clear from putrid wastes. Most people know this already and it's the reason why, for at least the last 30 years, 'eat more fibre' has been at the top of the healthy-things-to-do list. However, more recent research proves that this very special food category has much more to offer than merely a talent for swabbing and sweeping our personal sewage department! Many of the benefits can now be linked to the positive effects that different types of fibres (and especially the prebiotic variety) have on our gut bugs.

Defining fibre

Dietary fibre is found only in foods of plant origin: cereals, fruits, pulses (peas, beans and lentils), seeds, nuts, vegetables and wholegrains are rich in fibre. Fruit juices and vegetable juices are still a useful source of fibre if they contain some or all the original pulp, but not so much if they're processed or made using an extractor that takes out the fleshy bits. Refined grains, such as those used to produce white flour, have little or no fibre. Animal-sourced foods such as meat, fish, milk, eggs, butter and cheese contain none.

Fibre for different tasks

You may already know that there are two main types of fibre. One is called insoluble, meaning that it's not able to absorb water; the other is soluble, indicating that it does dissolve in water. This doesn't mean that one type of fibre is better than another. Nor does it follow that just because a food is listed as a valuable source of, say, soluble fibre, it doesn't contain insoluble fibre too. Nearly all plants have some of both kinds, but some have more soluble or more insoluble fibre. They're both essential for good health; it's just that they do different tasks. There's also another important category of fibre called resistant starch, which I'll be looking at later on.

The term 'fibre' is about as misleading as the old name 'roughage'. The main reason why insoluble fibre once upon a time had this tag is because, if you think about it, some of it does appear quite rough, tough and stringy. But many so-called 'fibres' are not actually fibrous at all; in fact, a lot of them are more like gum or gel. Take a nectarine, a plum or an aubergine as examples: the skin is made up of insoluble fibre and the fleshy inside contains mostly soluble fibre.

Why both are necessary

For the purposes of our health, it doesn't matter whether the actual fibrous parts resemble jelly or jute as long as we make sure we consume both types. The common denominator is that, even though the fruit or vegetable or grain they come from is edible, the soluble and insoluble fibre – found in leaves, roots, stalks, stems, skin, pips, seeds or pulp – pass through to the large intestine without being digested. This is what gives them their special attributes.

Insoluble fibre is the one that provides a plant with its structure, and is the type that's famous for keeping us 'regular'. Probably the best known of all roughage is the wheat bran so familiar of breakfast cereals. Other sources include brown rice, nuts, wheatgerm, wholemeal pasta, wholegrain flour, wholegrain bread, whole rye, fruits and vegetables, especially the skins and seeds. Although it can't actually absorb water, insoluble fibre does have a characteristic that attracts water to it. This is crucial for bulking and softening the stools so that they don't hang around where the sun doesn't shine and can travel more easily and quickly to the outside world!

Soluble fibre is predominant in foods such as pulses, vegetables, all kinds of fresh and dried fruits, oats, oat bran, whole oat flour, wholegrain and milled barley, rye, seeds and flax (linseed). Even though it isn't digested, soluble fibre does change its structure as it goes through a process of fermentation in the colon where it's broken down into a jelly-like mass. Soluble fibres are especially helpful at improving diabetic control, reducing fats in the blood, and increasing mineral absorption, especially calcium, iron and magnesium. And don't forget that many soluble fibres also have prebiotic qualities, which means that they're an important source of food for our good gut bugs, who use it to produce more friendly flora.

Resistant starch, so-called because it resists digestion, is a type of fibre found in wholegrains such as oats, some fruits, including bananas, in lentils and other pulses and some vegetables. It's referred to as the third type of dietary fibre, because some of it behaves like soluble fibre (it's fermented in the gut by bacteria), while the rest has the qualities of the bulking insoluble fibre. Resistant starch is also formed when foods that contain starch cool down after cooking. Examples of this are bread, cold pasta and cold, cooked potatoes (think pasta or potato salad).

In more detail ...
Because there are also plenty of other foods with prebiotic activity that are not 'fibrous' at all, such as yoghurt, goat's milk and raw honey, the official definition of dietary fibre has been expanded to include not only obviously fibrous foods but also any others that have a proven prebiotic action.

Super fibre

Fibre is important for several reasons:

- It helps to balance glucose levels in the blood and prevent any sudden or dramatic rise or fall of blood sugar; that's why high-fibre diets can be so valuable for diabetics and those suffering hypoglycaemia.

- The same mechanism maintains our energy levels by releasing energy slowly into the system after a meal. Quick fixes, like chocolate bars or cakes, release their sugars rapidly, which is why you can feel empty, tired and brain-fogged very quickly after eating them (and craving for more!).
- Dietary fibre grabs hold of and deactivates carcinogens, thereby reducing the risk of colon cancer.

Fibre can also:

- Protect against haemorrhoids, varicose veins, diverticular disease, gallstones, kidney disease and constipation.
- Keep you regular by speeding up the transit time of wastes through the gut.
- Reduce the build-up of toxins, yeasts and pathogenic bacteria.
- Stabilise blood fats and cholesterol.
- Improve the take-up and absorption of minerals, especially magnesium.

And be a valuable dietary support for people trying to lose weight.

How much fibre do I need every day?

Recommendations for the amounts of fibre you need vary widely depending on which country in the world you live in and which organisation you turn to for information; for example, in the UK, the minimum fibre intake for adults has been set at 18g per day (the average intake at the moment is only 12g). In the United States, 19g and 38g daily are the minimum and maximum figures. Australia pitches much higher at 35–45g. If you really need to know how much fibre a particular food contains, there are plenty of tables, books and charts available in libraries and on the Internet. And all packaged foods must tell you how much fibre is included in the product, so it's really worth becoming an avid label reader. However, if you follow the tips at the end of this chapter, you should be taking on board more than adequate amounts without needing to count anything.

> **!** **Very important point**
> Suddenly making big changes to your diet could make you a bit gassy or gripey, as the gut adjusts to its healthier intake. This is normal and the side effects are usually only very short term, but it's always best to go slowly at first.

Remember: don't eat wheat

I've talked about wheat products in the Good Gut Upgrade on page 44, but I mention it again here simply because many people are unaware that it is such a troublesome food. Wholewheat and wheat fibre can be a valuable fibre source for some people, but in others this type of coarse fibre can irritate the gut and especially the ileocaecal valve, which can then allow unwanted bacteria to backflow from the large to the small intestine. Experience shows that, for some, wheat-based foods can cause more problems than they solve. One major reason is that we eat too much of the stuff.

Wheat overload

If your diet regularly includes bread, toast, sandwiches, biscuits, wheat muesli, wheat-bran crackers, cakes, pastry, pasta, pies, pizza bases, and sauces or gravies that are made with flour, you could find yourself eating some kind of wheat-based food at almost every meal. As you will have seen from my chart at the end of Chapter 2, many people rely rather too heavily on white bread and highly refined white-flour products. But even if you're not one of them, you might still find that high-fibre wheat doesn't suit you too well. We're all encouraged to believe that wholegrain wheat is a good way to increase our intake of dietary fibre, and so it is, but there are a few things to watch out for.

First of all, wheat can hamper weight loss and cause discomfort and bloating. In addition, wheat-bran fibre, especially that found in breakfast cereals mentioned above, is high in a substance known as phytic acid, which, if taken in large amounts, can have a negative effect on the absorption of vitamin B_3 (niacin) and certain minerals from the diet. You should be aware of this if you eat a lot of this type of fibre. Interestingly, some of our friendly bacteria, including *Lactobacillus acidophilus*, help us to produce an enzyme called phytase, which helps to break down the phytic acid and make it more soluble (and less troublesome).

Sensitive systems beware

Take care, too, if you have a sensitive system. Wheat fibre is still recommended by most doctors and dieticians as a useful dietary fibre, even though it can be extremely unkind to a tender intestine. I find that many patients are puzzled when they have taken this kind of advice and increased their intake of this kind of fibre only to find themselves coping with a flare up of diverticular disease, IBS or piles and, in some cases, worsening constipation.

In the particular instance of irritable bowel syndrome, there's good evidence that, although a high-fibre diet can help, wheat-based foods are not always the best choice. As I explain to my own patients, if you're wheat-sensitive, using bran as your main source of roughage is a bit like expecting something with all the smoothness and charisma of a ball of Velcro to pass snag-free down the length of a 28-foot nylon stocking. Not the kind of thing you want if your gut is already a bit grouchy. Unfortunately for us wheat-sensitive souls, it often sneaks into products without you realising it's there, so if you're trying to steer clear of it, read every label. And be comforted by the fact that there are much better options available. See below.

Delicious alternatives to wheat

Instead of relying on wheat, why not consider oats, whole rice crackers or rice cakes, porridge, oat muesli, oatcakes, buckwheat crackers, brown basmati rice, rye bread and Ryvita crispbread? The less well-known grains such as quinoa or kamut also make great – and very healthy – options. It may take a bit of sleuthing in specialist markets, delicatessens or health-food stores but the effort is really worth it for the sake of your good gut bugs. Thankfully, many of the major supermarkets are now beginning to cater for people who prefer to avoid wheat.

Even then, don't rely totally on cereals for your daily quota. We need other kinds of fibre too, in particular from fruit and vegetables. That's another reason why it is really worth aiming for that minimum five-a-day.

Soothing psyllium

Psyllium comes from the family of plants known as *Plantago* and contains both kinds of fibre but more insoluble than soluble. The reason why the seeds and husks are so beneficial is because they're incredibly gentle on the gut. Like all good fibre, psyllium bulks the stool and eases the passage of waste through the large colon. It's also considered a valuable natural, drug-free, internal cleanser and has, like milled flaxseed, an adaptogenic and regulatory action that makes it equally useful for the treatment of diarrhoea, constipation, diverticulitis, haemorrhoids and irritable bowel syndrome. In clinical studies approved by the US Food and Drug Administration, the soluble fibre in psyllium is shown to lower cholesterol. There is evidence, too, that it may have anti-inflammatory properties.

Psyllium – also called isphagula – is sometimes included in prescription and over-the-counter fibre products and, in some countries, is added to breakfast cereals. Interestingly, I've had many patients tell me that prescription isphagula doesn't suit them, causing griping and bloating, especially in ultra-sensitive intestines, whereas ordinary plain psyllium appears to be much better tolerated. So perhaps there's an additive or some kind of different processing in the prescription version that upsets a tetchy gut? Natural psyllium is a worthwhile alternative, especially for anyone with bowel disorders such as IBS. Your independent health-food store should stock psyllium-based products. Always take psyllium with lots of water.

Max on the flax

Psyllium has many benefits, but flaxseed (also known as linseed) is often regarded as unequalled when it comes to quality fibre; perhaps because there's a better balance of soluble and insoluble fibre, which means that some of it is fermented by the intestinal bacteria, acting as prebiotic support for our good gut bugs, while the rest of it goes for bulk. Quality flax fibre also contains lignans[JB].

Jargon buster

Lignans are a group of protective plant nutrients that not only have strong antioxidant properties but also contain phytoestrogens – best known for helping to ease the symptoms of the menopause, but also being studied as an important possible defence in the fight against certain types of cancer.

Lignans are found in grains, pulses, vegetables and seeds – in particular oats, soya beans, broccoli, cabbage, sesame seeds and pumpkin seeds – berry fruits, good red wine and, especially, flaxseed, which is nature's richest known source. Research shows that these important substances could reduce the risk of heart and circulatory disorders, cholesterol levels and cancers, not only of the colon but also of the breast and prostate, as well as giving possible improvements in diabetes, skin disorders and bone density. They're really important, too, in helping to reduce inflammation, which can be part and parcel of a long list of unpleasant diseases (see Chapter 24).

The level of lignans in good-quality flax is useful but not always high. Where lignans are recommended in therapeutic doses for certain conditions, you may be advised to go for a concentrated lignan supplement such as Estrolignan from Bionutri or Viridian 100% Organic Golden Flaxseed Oil, which is also a great vegetarian alternative to omega-3 fish oil supplements.

One of the best favours you could do for yourself is to add flax fibre to your daily routine and to regard it as a regular food.

It's gentle and kind to the gut, and nudges the most reluctant bowel into moving wastes along the tube to where we all know they should be: down the toilet.

For best results, follow these important points:

1 Ignore cheap brands and buy the best that you can afford. The better ones will be vacuumed sealed. Flaxseed is very susceptible to contamination by daylight, heat and air, which degrades the special oils that it contains, so avoid any brands that are sold loose or in regular see-through or non-vacuum packaging. If you come across linseed/flaxseed, either milled or whole, which seems to be a real bargain, the chances are that it won't be. Even if the seed was of good quality to begin with, the oils are probably degraded, which means that they won't be good for you.

2 Some people prefer to buy whole seed because they say that it's less likely to have degraded than seed that is already milled. And of course you can grind the seed yourself as and when you need it. But this only applies if the seed is top quality to begin with and, in any event, I know a lot of people who reckon they only just about make time to swallow their breakfast, never mind finding extra valuable minutes to grind up seeds every morning. Another thing to keep in mind is that whole seeds may not be suitable for some people with a very sensitive gut or who have been advised by their doctor to avoid seeded foods. My personal preference is for quality vacuum-sealed organic milled seed, which I find very helpful for people with conditions such as irritable bowel syndrome, diverticular disease, Crohn's disease or ulcerative colitis.

3 Remember that if you add flaxseed to hot food or use it in baking, you will still get the beneficial fibre but will have 'corrupted' and spoiled the valuable oils.

Which brands are best?

These are the ones I usually recommend:

- **Linwoods Organic Milled Flaxseed** is widely available throughout the UK and Europe. It can be found in independent health-food stores and via the Internet. Prices vary widely, so shop around before deciding. For more information, go to www.linwoods.co.uk. If you buy elsewhere, check that you're getting *milled* flaxseed before you checkout.

- **Linusit Gold** is good-quality whole seed, available from health-food stores and some supermarkets. You can swallow the whole seed if you want to – they are very small and slide down easily. But you won't get the same benefits as you would from grinding the seed or soaking it first.

- **Linoforce** is a product based on linseeds but, in this case, has added senna, a traditional plant remedy that can be especially helpful if bowels are really sluggish. This is a useful product for anyone suffering constipation that doesn't seem to respond to other treatments. I have used it very successfully in elderly patients with resistant constipation and also for people with diverticular disease. If you've had all the tests and been given a clean bill of health but are still suffering, try this product for a month. It's also the one to choose if you're recovering from surgery for haemorrhoids (see page 205) when every bowel movement feels like passing broken glass. Do bear in mind that a little Linoforce goes a very long way, so try half a teaspoon per day to begin with and increase by a quarter teaspoon until an easy bowel movement is achieved. Because of the senna content being so laxative, it's not advised that you use Linoforce long term unless you have discussed the dosage with your doctor. If you're pregnant, use it only with medical supervision. Never exceed the stated amount and don't take it at the same time as other laxative preparations. More information is available from www.avogel.co.uk. Once you're back to normal, ease up on the Linoforce and change to the Linwood product (above). Or check out your independent health-food store, or search online, for other top-quality milled flaxseed products.

Did you know?

Research shows that non-vegetarians have lower amounts of those all-important lignan substances in their blood than vegetarians who, by the way, also have fewer cancers than meat eaters. Although it isn't saying that people who prefer not to be vegetarian have to give up eating animal-sourced foods to be healthy, it does confirm the importance of upping the intake of vegetables, pulses, nuts and seeds.

A note about oils

When we talk about linseed oil, most people think of the stuff that we use to treat wood. This is not nutritional linseed or flaxseed oil. So what about the flaxseed oil you can buy in the health-food store, which is often favoured by people who suffer with dry skin or sore joints? If it's the best quality, sold in a properly sealed, opaque container and from organic sources, it will probably be rich in nutritious substances known as essential fatty acids. But non-organic oils or those in clear bottles won't contain much, if any, worthwhile goodness.

How to take flaxseed/linseed fibre

It's important to begin with a low dose so, whatever the pack instructions say, I would suggest starting with only one teaspoon of powder or seed with a decent-sized glass of water first thing in the morning. Going slowly and working up to a full daily dose gives your body the chance to adjust. After a few days, increase your daily intake to two teaspoonfuls and then, after a couple of weeks, perhaps to three teaspoons but always remember the importance of the water. Even though it's OK to add to food, the risk is that you won't drink enough water with it, simply because your appetite is satisfied and you may not feel you have enough room. So do make sure that you always include a large glass of water with your meal, or take your flaxseed and water together first thing in the morning. Water is vital in order for the fibre to work properly.

Do you need to take fibre supplements?

If you follow the advice in this chapter there should be no need to take fibre in the form of capsules. However, they can be useful in certain circumstances; for example, if you're going to be away from home, in hospital or on holiday – all situations where the bowels can be temporarily temperamental – then fibre supplements are easy to pack and simple to take. You might choose a brand that contains just fibre, or a better alternative could be to go for those that contain psyllium together with other ingredients such as barberry bark, burdock root, clove, garlic, slippery elm and bentonite clay, all excellent ingredients for a sluggish colon. These 'extras' are also valuable in cases of stubborn constipation where, occasionally, even the most fibrous diet won't shift the waste. Remember that the same advice about fluid intake applies here. Never use fibre supplements without drinking plenty of water.

There are lots of really good products on the market from reliable companies such as Sunshine Health Shop, Natural Dispensary, NutriGold, Viridian Nutrition, Higher Nature, Biocare, G&G Foods, Victoria Health, Solgar and Arkopharma. NutriGold Colon Support Formula is a particular favourite of mine because of the positive feedback that I get from patients who use it (see Resources).

Kathryn's top ten fibre tips

Here are a few more tips on upping your fibre intake. By copying at least some of the suggestions here, you'll not only be adding to your intake of important prebiotic foods but you'll also be getting closer to the recommended five fruit and vegetable servings. And, in the process, you'll be increasing your intake of a whole range of important nutrients.

1 Widen your horizons! Don't fall into the trap of limiting yourself to just a few familiar favourites. This is really important because the most beneficial effects are likely to come from including combinations of different prebiotic and fibrous foods. Every time you go to the grocery store, market or supermarket, why not try a different vegetable or fruit that you haven't tried before? Frozen fruits and vegetables still contain worthwhile dietary fibre and are good standbys when fresh equivalents are unavailable.

2 Add extras to your lunch. Go beyond cucumber, tomato and iceberg; think about adding avocado pear, beansprouts, beetroot, grated carrot and dark leaf lettuce. Sprinkle a few sunflower, sesame or pumpkin seeds over. Remember that fresh herbs can lift a salad from the ordinary to the extraordinary. If the weather seems too chilly for salad on its own, why not eat it alongside a hot dish such as home-made vegetable soup, a jacket potato or brown rice and beans.

3 Make fresh vegetable soup, then it's available for lunch or for putting into a flask for taking to work. Even if you don't like vegetables or you don't like to cook, it's the easiest thing in the world to throw some carrot, onion, garlic, broccoli (especially the stalks), butternut squash, parsnip and potato into a pan, simmer until tender, then blend into a smooth soup. This mix is filling, nourishing, incredibly tasty, cheap to produce and loaded with important prebiotics.

4 Add an extra vegetable to your main meal of the day. Most people who say they don't like vegetables will still manage to eat potatoes and peas but, although there's nothing wrong with either of these foods, sticking with the same few favourites means your diet could be lacking in variety and some essential vitamins and minerals.

5 Try to include one or two pieces of fresh fruit – or one piece of fruit and a fresh juice – every day. It's worth a reminder that, although juice extractors may seem like a great idea, you're losing out on a considerable quantity of valuable fibre. One way around this is to mix back some of the pulp into the juice before you drink it or, do as we do at home, forget the juicer and just dump chopped fruit into a blender. Even if you discard the peel, you'll still get all that really healthy soluble fibre from the soft pulp. Just add some water so that the blender blades turn smoothly. Another plus point here is that you can 'lose' two pieces of fruit into one juice drink and straight away you've achieved two of your daily minimum of five servings.

6 Use plenty of pulses. Add beans and lentils to soups, casseroles and salads. Try original baked beans (not low cal) as a filling snack. Make hummus paste with chickpeas, garlic and olive oil. Include foods from the list of fibre providers on page 103. Stock the store cupboard with canned pulses, and chuck them into all kinds of dishes. A tin of butter beans, chickpeas or lentils, rinsed thoroughly and whizzed in a blender, makes a fabulously healthy thickener for soups, sauces and gravies.

7 Potatoes are a great fibre source. How about a delicious potato salad with chopped fried onion, chopped chives and a splash of dressing made with extra virgin olive oil? Don't forget that cold cooked potatoes are rich in a different kind of fibre called resistant starch. Or choose sweet potatoes for a nutritious change.

If possible, buy organic potatoes (new or old), and eat them in their skins. What about ordinary non-organic spuds? Well, it's up to you. I prefer not to eat the skins because I'm concerned about the sprays that are used.

8 Instead of biscuits, cakes, chocolate and crisps, snack on fibre-rich foods such as sunflower and pumpkin seeds, carrots, apples, small amounts of dried fruit and, unless you're allergic to them, Brazil nuts, almonds and walnuts.

9 Make your own breakfast cereal. Oats not only make great porridge but they're also a wonderful prebiotic food to use as a base for home-made muesli. Add chopped nuts, seeds and dried fruit, plus a spoonful of plain full-fat (yes, full fat!) Greek yoghurt for a healthy, sustaining breakfast. Or soak dried fruit such as apricots, prunes and figs, and serve with yoghurt for fabulous fibre, plenty of nutrients and a sweet treat all in the same bowl.

10 Up your intake of water. Yes, I know that water isn't fibrous, but I've included it in this top ten list because it's vital in helping your body to process your new high-fibre prebiotic diet.

Take care
Don't give flaxseed or psyllium to children under five years of age. That's because an infant gut hasn't matured sufficiently to cope with excess amounts. That doesn't mean that they can't handle or don't need dietary fibre, but care should be taken not to overload an immature digestive system with high intakes of insoluble fibre and to ensure that they're given enough sugar-free fluids, preferably water.

> Elderly people who aren't used to fibre should also be cautious. In later life, narrowing of the large intestine, reduced mobility, lack of fluid intake, poor diet or poor digestion can reduce the body's ability to cope with large amounts of fibre, which could cause compaction, blockage, severe pain and even death.
>
> If a very young or elderly person is constipated, it's best to consult the doctor or practice nurse before attempting to give laxatives or additional dietary fibre.

Which foods for fibre?

There are so many good sources of dietary fibre that can be relied upon to do their thing. In alphabetical order, here are just a few:

Almonds
Apples
Apricots – fresh or dried
Artichokes
Asparagus
Aubergines
Bananas
Barley
Beetroot
Black-eyed peas
Blackberries
Blueberries
Broccoli
Brown rice
Brussels sprouts
Buckwheat (not related to ordinary wheat)
Butter beans
Cabbage
Cannellini beans
Carrots
Cauliflower
Celery
Chickpeas
Chicory
Coconut

Cold cooked potatoes
Coleslaw
Courgette
Dried fruit (small amounts)
Figs – fresh or dried
Flaxseed (linseed)
Garlic
Green beans
Haricot beans
Hummus (chickpea paste)
Jacket potato
Jícama (Mexican potato)
Leeks
Lentils
Lima beans
Kamut
Kiwi fruit
Mango
Nuts
Oats
Onions
Papaya
Peaches
Pears
Peas
Potatoes in skins

Prunes
Pulses
Pumpkin seeds
Quinoa
Raisins
Raspberries
Red kidney beans
Rice cakes
Rice pasta
Rye bread
Ryvita crackers
Sesame seeds
Snow peas/sugar snaps

Spelt flour
Spelt pasta
Spinach
Spring onions
Sultanas
Sunflower seeds
Sweet potatoes
Tomatoes
Walnuts
Whole barley
Whole rye
Yacón (root vegetable)

Snippet

One of the most fibrous fruits available is said to be the Amazonian palm berry. Between 25 and 50 per cent of its content is fibre.

7.

Antibiotics – Friend or Foe?

❛Bacteria keep us from heaven and (also) put us there. ❜

Martin Henry Fischer 1879–1962, Professor of physiology at the University of Cincinnati, famous for his book of sayings called *Fischerisms*

Everybody should read this chapter!

I'd like to begin this chapter by telling you a really interesting story. In the 1830s, two young chemists called John May and William Garrard Baker formed a company, May & Baker. This isn't a name that's likely to be familiar to every reader, but older generations may recognise it and know why it is justifiably famous. In the beginning, they produced chemical ingredients for sale to pharmaceutical companies, and later they also manufactured medicines, their first being a sedative called Sulphonal. In 1936/7 research chemists in May & Baker's Dagenham factory developed a product that was so innovative, so incredibly important and needed so urgently that they didn't even waste time thinking up a name for it, so they referred to it by its production code M&B 693.

The company's fame spread on the back of this one product because it was the first cure for a disease that, up to this point, had been a killer: bacterial pneumonia.

Because of the significance of the May & Baker discovery being made just before the Second World War, and for the reason that M&B drugs were suddenly needed in such large quantities, medical production was put on to a war footing. Other sulphonamides (also known as sulphur drugs), in particular the M&B 760, were soon to follow. But M&B 693 holds the prize for the first available antibacterial. It was the forerunner of antibiotics and preceded penicillin's actual manufacture by several years.

> ### Snippet
> I have a very personal reason to be grateful to M&B 693. When my husband Richard was a very small boy he contracted bacterial pneumonia and was so ill that he wasn't expected to live. The doctor called to see the patient and took along with him a sample of this new drug, so new that it didn't even have a proper container. 'It has to be worth a try,' he told Richard's mother, 'because there's nothing else available and nothing else we can do.' It worked, and Richard made a full recovery. He keeps esteemed company when it comes to M&B 693:
>
> When Winston Churchill fell ill in Carthage, Tunisia in 1943, and was suspected of having pneumonia, his physician administered M&B 693. On 29 December 1943, he told the British nation in wonderful Churchillian tones: 'This admirable "M&B" from which I did not suffer any inconvenience was used at the earliest moment and after a week's fever the intruders were repulsed.'

Mouldy business

Although it's usually Alexander Fleming who gets the credit for discovering penicillin (around 1928), he really wasn't the first. More than 30 years earlier, Ernest Duchesne, at the time a medic in the French army, noticed how Arab stable lads in North Africa used a particular mould to treat their horses' saddle sores.

Many other ancient cultures, including Russian, Egyptian, Greek, Serbian and Sri Lankan, had long been aware that moulds could take care of infections even though they probably didn't know why it worked. Three thousand years ago, the Chinese covered boils and skin infections with mouldy soya bean curd and, throughout history, poultices have been made from mouldy bread or mouldy cake to treat battlefield wounds.

Fast forward to 1898 where, after some detailed experiments, Dr Duchesne identified his mould as being *Penicillium glaucum* and proved its worth by using it to bump off a whole load of pathogenic *E. coli* bacteria. He also did some studies using guinea pigs (real ones, not coerced humans) and showed that this particular mould could wipe out typhoid. He submitted his findings in his doctoral thesis to the Pasteur Institute in Paris – who ignored it completely.

Sadly, this momentous breakthrough sunk into oblivion when, in 1912, poor Ernest popped off the planet, having succumbed to tuberculosis. The irony here is that the cure for his disease would later be found to be …? Yes, penicillin.

Developments in the 20th century

Another generally disregarded milestone came in 1923 when André Gratia, a Belgian researcher working in molecular biology and bacteriology, was studying the behaviour of pathogenic bacteria and noticed that a mould had contaminated one of the dishes of a bug known as *Staphylococcus aureus*, slowing up the bacterial growth. He realised that it was a type of *Penicillium* and presented his findings, which were also pretty much ignored. At around the same time, a Nicaraguan-born scientist and prolific researcher who gloried in the name of Clodomiro Picado Twight, was working at the Pasteur Institute when he recorded that *Penicillium* mould had an antibacterial effect. As a result of his laboratory work he went on to use it successfully to treat his patients.

All of this was happening at least a year before Alexander Fleming shouted 'Got it!' Although he gets the Brownie points for coming up with the name 'penicillin', in truth he didn't discover it. He may have 're-discovered' it, but he certainly wasn't the sole creator, and the accolades that have been heaped upon him are said by several historians to be entirely disproportionate to his contribution.

Penicillin saves lives on the battlefield

Another ten years were to pass before major research into the use of penicillin as an antibiotic would be advanced by the Oxford team of Howard Florey, Ernst Boris Chain and Norman Heatley from 1939 and into the early years of the war. Without their persistence and determination, its further development might never have taken place. By D-Day, it was being dispatched to field hospitals. With the availability of easily applied penicillin dressings, the chance of a wound getting infected was vastly curtailed and survival rates greatly increased. It's astonishing how this one drug so dramatically reduced the number of amputations, which had been so common-place during the First World War.

The success of penicillin and the M&B medications triggered a massive explosion of research into new products, including more and different antibiotics, and formed the basis of the modern pharmaceutical industry that we know today. It's impossible to say how many lives have been saved as a result of the pre-war work on bacteria-busting drugs, but several sources at the time of writing estimate several hundred million.

The downsides

The first snag of antibiotics and one that almost everyone must have experienced at some time or another is side effects. All pharmaceutical medicines have them. Some people are affected a lot, others less so, and a few lucky souls not at all. Some drugs produce more bad reactions than others. We accept these unpleasant symptoms as part of the treatment, because we hope the medication will cure us. When it comes to antibiotics, there are a few I'm sure you'll know about. If you didn't get 'the runs', you might have leaned in the other direction and ended up with constipation. Or maybe you were really bloated and uncomfortable, or you lost your sense of taste. Or perhaps you felt sick or actually threw up? And when you finished the course, you weren't out of the woods, because you got thrush or some other fungal infection? Or perhaps you were lucky and didn't notice any unpleasant effects at all?

Severe reactions

Some people are severely allergic to antibiotics, most commonly to penicillin. Symptoms can include skin rashes and, more danger-ously, problems with breathing and swelling of the mouth, tongue and face. This is called anaphylaxis and it can be fatal. If that's you, you'll probably already know it and your medical file should have a note written somewhere in plain sight so that there's almost no risk of anyone giving you penicillin. But never assume that the nurse or doctor, pharmacist or paramedic who is dealing with you already knows about your allergy. Tell them just in case. Another safety measure is to wear a Medic-Alert tag or bracelet or to carry an emergency-warning card in your wallet or purse.

Unsuitable partners

There are several medicines that can either interfere with the effectiveness of the antibiotic itself or that may not be so helpful if they're taken alongside antibiotics. Unwise combinations of certain drugs could also have unpleasant adverse effects. So, if you're on any kind of regular or temporary medication, whether it's prescribed or bought from the pharmacy, and you have to take antibiotics as well, then tell your doctor and/or pharmacist. This applies particularly to some antihistamines and some herbal medicines.

Certain types of antibiotic can affect the contraceptive pill, meaning that it might not work. If you were unlucky enough to have diarrhoea while you were on antibiotics, it's possible that you might not have absorbed your contraceptive pill properly. If you were actually sick, you may have ejected it. Apart from needing to consider alternative protection, please also make sure you talk to your doctor or pharmacist about any drug interactions.

Another major downside

Every success holds within itself the seeds of its own destruction, and unfortunately this is also true of antibiotic medication. The particular negative that I'm talking about here is, of course, antibiotic resistance. Doctors and scientists call it antimicrobial resistance and it simply means the ability of bacteria to withstand – or resist – the effects of antibiotic treatment.

Why don't antibiotics work so well anymore?

Say an opportunist bug finds its way into the body and, as a result, we get an infection. Most times the immune system will chase it out or kill it off. But where resistance is low, or when the body is confronted with an overwhelming number of invaders, there are occasions when it simply can't cope. The choice we now face is to allow these vast quantities of unwanted bacteria to multiply to the point where they make us ill or to call on antibiotics to destroy the invading bacteria.

Over the years since antibiotics became widely available, they were seen as such miracle medicines that they were often prescribed for conditions that didn't need them; for example, viruses, such as colds, which don't respond to these drugs. That's because antibiotics only deal with bacteria. It also used to be commonplace for doctors to recommend antibiotics on what was known as a 'just-in-case' basis – in case the patient with the cold developed a hacking cough or a raging chest infection or 'strep' throat, even if there was no evidence for it at that particular moment.

Keeping the luxury

'Most of us are either still alive or have family members who are still alive because an antibiotic conquered an infectious disease that otherwise would have killed the individual. If we want to retain this medical luxury in our society we must be vigilant and proactive . . . we must maintain a stride ahead of pathogens.'
Dr Stephen Abedon, Department of Microbiology, Ohio State University.

Disturbing the balance

When we take antibiotics, the hope is that they beat the bacteria that caused the infection and we get better. But whether they're used properly or taken unnecessarily, they will, without doubt, disturb the delicate balance of bacteria in our bodies, irritating the intestines and altering the levels of gut flora. Repeated use of antibiotics can result in a condition known as dysbiosis, a disturbance of friendly bacteria that leads to overgrowth of pathogens, which, in turn, can trigger a long list of other health problems.

Although it's now recognised by doctors and patients alike that antibiotics have been horribly overused, the realisation has dawned too late to prevent the emergence of certain types and strains of bacteria evolving with a particularly unpleasant personality trait: the ability to survive antibiotic treatment.

What causes antibiotic resistance?

Antibiotic resistance happens when a drug that was originally designed to kill bacteria is no longer effective. That's why the search is on to find new treatments that can deal with what are known as antibiotic-resistant bacterial strains, such as the superbugs we know as MRSA and *Clostridium difficile*. (See Chapter 8 for the Scary Story of Superbugs.)

So why are so many antibiotics no longer capable of doing the job they were originally designed for? First of all, antibiotics are effectively blind. They go in with guns blazing, unable to discriminate between good bacteria and bad. The good thing is that this broad-spectrum activity is more likely to wipe out unidentified pathogens, but the bad news is that broad-spectrum antibiotics also wipe out the good guys that are there to protect us. This weakens our defences and leaves the way clear for pathogenic bacteria to thrive. And these bad bacteria are smart. They're always one step ahead.

Survival instinct

Throughout evolution bad bacteria have been extremely clever at adapting constantly to their environment and taking on the personality of other bacteria. When antibiotics are used too often or unnecessarily, even though they might still manage to kill off some of the weaker germs, they'll often leave the stronger ones alive and thriving. Once the bad bacteria have managed to resist one type of antibiotic, they're better equipped to resist others. They learn to protect themselves by swapping genetic material between each other and then, once they've taken on board several resistant genes, they get promoted and can officially call themselves multi-resistant bacteria, otherwise known as superbugs.

What we have done

Unwittingly, we've made matters worse by:

- Taking antibiotics when it's not necessary or when they're inappropriately prescribed – such as for cold viruses or for nonbacterial bladder problems.

- Following repeated courses of antibiotics, especially for skin conditions or recurring bladder infections when there are better and safer forms of treatment available that don't disturb the gut flora.

- Being given the wrong antibiotic for the condition concerned.

- Failing to take a vital antibiotic prescription according to the dosage instructions; for example, not completing the course, even though it's something that's emphasised over and over by medics and pharmacists alike.

- Consuming foods that contain antibiotic residues. The development of antibiotic-resistant bacteria has also been compounded by the disproportionate use of antibiotics in farming, in particular to promote growth. Eating food products (especially meat, dairy and poultry) that carry antibiotic residues from animals means that we ingest them into our digestive systems, a bit like a drip feed, a little at a time, drip, drip, drip. Fruit can also be a problem where trees or bushes have been treated with sprays containing antibiotics.

And think on this: when we empty our bladders (or our bowels), those residues pass into the sewage system and eventually into the water table where they're taken up by other creatures, including fish and farm animals. Round and round we go. There's plenty of evidence of antibiotics being found in drinking water supplies in various parts of the world. And all the while, this is ideal ammunition for pathogenic bacteria who never give up trying to find new ways to resist.

? Did you know?
The United States alone produces 35 million pounds in weight (just short of 16 million kilos) of antibiotics every year and at least half of this is used in animals. The most worrying aspect is that the majority of these drugs (around 80 per cent of that half) are targeted, specifically, at encouraging weight gain in animal livestock.

Increasingly, however, probiotics are being added to animal feedstuffs and, as a result, could have significant benefits for human health. Such a move may also be better for farm animals generally by helping to strengthen their resistance to infectious diseases.

Second-hand antibiotics

The result of all this is that we've unwittingly created what experts call a reservoir of antibiotic-resistant bacteria and much of that resistance is now developing not only in people who are taking the antibiotics but also in the wider environment. Even if someone isn't exposed to antibiotic residues (although it's unlikely that they won't at some stage in their lives), there's the additional risk of being attacked by bacteria that have already come into contact with antibiotics and so are already drug-resistant. The chilling aspect is that there is now a danger of exposure to what are being tagged 'second-hand antibiotics'.

Let's look at a couple of studies. In one, patients who were treated with an antibiotic called erythromycin developed skin bacteria that were found to be resistant to the drug (no surprise there). But the body blow for scientists was to discover that other people in the same house also showed similar resistance, *even though they themselves were not taking the antibiotics!* In an investigation along similar lines, chickens fed low doses of antibiotics developed resistance within only a couple of weeks and then passed on that resistance to the farm workers, *even though the workers themselves were not taking antibiotics!* The problem is being made worse by the fact that we are now swamping our surroundings with megatons of antibacterial cleaning and washing products, all of which are having a devastating global impact and making it easier, not harder, for pathogenic bacteria to gain the upper hand.

What can we do about it?

The gloom and doom merchants predict that the likely outcome is probably not a nice one. Some ghastly superbug will eventually rear up in a real-life replay of a disaster movie and wipe us all out at a stroke so that, in the final scene, the only human still standing is Will Smith!

Why such pessimism? It's because resistance to antibiotics is still on the increase, a fact confirmed over and over by the number of reported cases of superbug outbreaks in hospitals around the UK that simply cannot be treated. Almost everyone you talk to has a horror story to tell about someone they know who has contracted MRSA or *C. difficile* or perhaps one of the other out-of-control superbugs and has either been desperately ill or has died. Vulnerable people, such as the elderly, and those with already compromised immune systems are more at risk, but these devastating infections can affect anyone – and not only in hospitals. Bacterial plagues are rampaging unseen through the community, too. No wonder the race is on to find an answer. But while the drug companies spend billions trying to develop new drugs that may – or may not – get us out of this sinister situation, we could be doing quite a lot to help ourselves.

For a start, we could use antibiotics more wisely:

1 Don't take them unless it's really necessary. Most people now accept that these drugs are not effective against everything, such as the aforementioned colds and flu. My own practice experience is that antibiotics aren't always helpful for urinary infections, ear infections or sinusitis either. And don't demand antibiotics for something that ails you just because you think you should have them or because someone you know was given them for a similar condition. What suits one person may not be appropriate for another.

2 Don't take antibiotics for extended periods of time unless you have a particular problem that really warrants such action and

you are under very regular medical review. Just recently I've been witness to two frightening cases of reckless use of antibiotics. One patient had been given them by her GP because of a history of cystitis and the other, by a different doctor, for acne. It wasn't the actual prescribing that was such a problem but the fact that both patients had been taking these drugs continuously (I mean every day!) over several years on a repeat prescription basis without any kind of consultation or check-up in between. Not surprisingly, both had developed serious bowel problems as a result of long-term damage to their gut microflora and were also suffering repeated chest infections because of reduced immunity. It's easy to forget that just because a particular drug has been found to be effective against a given bacterial infection or condition, it doesn't necessarily mean that it will remain so indefinitely.

3 If you live in a country where you can buy antibiotics direct from the pharmacy, get advice from the senior pharmacist on duty or see a doctor first. Specific bacterial infections may need specific drugs. Choosing any old antibiotic for whatever ails you could either be totally ineffective or dangerous.

4 If something is about to be prescribed, find out what type of antibiotic it is. First, check to make sure that it's the right one for your condition. Remember that not all antibiotics, even those with wide-ranging killing power, can inhibit all types of bacteria. Then ask if it's 'broad-spectrum': one that's designed to wipe out all bacteria. If yes, do you really need it or is there something better? Although annihilating everything might seem like a great way to hit the one that's causing the trouble, a broad-spectrum antibiotic can have a greater risk of long-term damage and adverse effects, because it isn't necessarily going to be aiming at the right target. Worse is the fact that broad-spectrum antibiotics can be death to all your good gut bugs, leaving you more susceptible to diarrhoea, thrush/candida yeast, superbugs and their complications, including *Clostridium difficile* colitis. If this wasn't enough to contemplate, there's also the risk of compromised immunity and the likelihood of yet further infections seeming to 'come from nowhere' almost the very second that the course of antibiotics is completed.

In the majority of cases, antibiotics are prescribed on what is known as a 'best guess' basis, the presumption being that in any type of infection there will be a shortlist of possible pathogenic perpetrators and, with it, an even shorter list of appropriate antibiotics that have a successful history in sorting out that particular condition. Because best guesses are hit and miss, the ideal is to delay the prescription and carry out laboratory tests to isolate the specific bacterium. Once a doctor has the result, he or she may then be able to recommend a narrow-spectrum antibiotic which fires directly at the pathogen concerned and has a less devastating effect on your body's friendly flora. The dilemma in all of this is deciding whether to risk an infection becoming worse while you wait for lab results or save time and tests (and sod the gut flora) by going in with broad-spectrum guns blazing.

Did you know?
Where antibiotics are essential, an approach the doctor may take is to prescribe two different antibiotics simultaneously. The reasoning behind this is based on the finding that, apart from doubling up the killing power, some bacteria may be less likely to develop resistance to two drugs than when just one drug is used on its own.

5 If you find that you do have to take antibiotics, follow the directions that are given to you by the doctor or the pharmacist or, if you're not sure, check the pack for dosage instructions.

6 Take the whole course. Stopping partway through, even if the symptoms seem to have disappeared, hugely racks up the risk of the infection returning, because, at the halfway stage, it's unlikely all of the bacteria will have been destroyed. Failing to complete the course also increases the likelihood of bacteria becoming resistant. And remember that it really isn't sensible to hoard pills for later use or to share prescriptions with anyone else.

7 If you do have any out-of-date or unused medication, take it back to your pharmacy. *Never* flush it down the toilet or into the washbasin. That's a surefire way of adding further antibiotic

residues to the water supply and to the sea. And don't leave it for the rubbish truck either; someone else, perhaps a child, a nosy pet or some vulnerable wildlife, might find it.

Reduce the risk of bacterial resistance

1 Keep surfaces clean, especially in bathrooms and food-preparation areas, but don't buy into the emotional blackmail that tells you you're irresponsible unless you use products that promise Apocalypse Now for all germs. There are plenty of excellent products based on organic ingredients and essential oils that do a perfectly good cleaning job without the devastation of modern chemical bug killers. A simple but strong solution of hot water and cider vinegar can dispatch most bacteria without disturbing the natural balance. In particular, avoid anything that contains Triclosan (an antibacterial agent) because bacteria are showing resistance against it. Research suggests that it might be toxic or damaging to humans in a number of other ways, too. For more information go to www.beyondpesticides.org, www.chemicalbodyburden.org and also www.ewg.org, which is the website for The Environmental Working Group.

2 There is some concern, too, about strong chemical-based antibacterial soaps and cleansers. These may be best kept for hospital use and for situations where someone is caring for a sick person who has been in hospital or who has weakened immunity. The daily onslaught of chemical cleansers we use on our skin, in the shower and on the hair could not only encourage bacteria to become resistant but may also disrupt the normal, good bacteria that help protect us both inside and outside the body.

3 There are plenty of environmentally friendly and organic products that are just as antimicrobial (they slow the growth of bacteria) without the devastating knock-on effects, so it's worth hunting for kinder alternatives. Although it's been widely reported that many of the big companies are beginning to use more natural ingredients, there are already some truly excellent eco-friendly products available from stores and online that are completely free of worrying ingredients. Find recommendations and more info in Resources on page 282.

4 Doctors and health-care professionals can help by:

- Isolating patients who succumb to drug-resistant infections.
- Being aware of the latest information concerning superbugs and antibiotic resistance.
- Not giving in to patient demands for antibiotics.
- Considering the use of two antibiotics at the same time. Research shows that treating with more than one drug simultaneously can kill more pathogens and could make it more difficult for a particular bacterium to become resistant.
- Prescribing broad-spectrum antibiotics only when absolutely necessary and preferentially using narrow-spectrum drugs that target a narrower range of bacteria.
- Washing hands thoroughly between seeing each patient, even if that patient has not been examined.
- Keeping an eye out for vitamin deficiencies. The devastating wipe-out of friendly flora that is caused by antibacterial drugs can also have an unseen yet detrimental effect on a range of nutrients. This lowers immunity and increases the risk of repeated infection and the need for yet more antibiotics.
- Recommending that probiotics are taken both during and after antibiotics.

Washing hands

There's no getting away from the fact that we don't wash our hands often enough. Research proves time and again the benefits to be gained by washing hands, at the very least after every visit to the bathroom, when caring for someone who is unwell, on returning from work or shopping, after playing with pets and, of course, always before preparing food.

There are plenty of gentle, but nonetheless effective, handwash alternatives. I like to use the Green People Organic Anti-bacterial Hand Wash or their Foaming Hand Sanitizer or the Quash Hand Sanitizer available from Big Green Smile. Also excellent is Maximum Strength Neem Oil Soap by Organix and Huni Propolis & Manuka soap, both available from Xynergy Health Products. Or you might like to try adding a few drops of tea tree or manuka oil to a plain liquid pH-balanced soap (see my note on page 136 about antibacterial oils). There is more on personal-care products in Resources.

> **Snippet**
> It's surprising how many people view hand washing as unnecessary. There have been several surveys carried out using hidden cameras, which show that the majority of people come straight out of the public toilet or the bathroom without bothering even to wave a cursory digit under the tap. They'll go to the loo, poke their ears, scratch their noses, touch doorknobs or trolley handles, and then, if you're really lucky, they'll make you a sandwich. Pretty amazingly, even those who do find the washbasin apparently don't know how to wash their hands properly.
>
> The recognised method is to soap not only the palms but also around and under the nails, over the backs of the hands and between the thumbs and fingers. Rinsing and drying thoroughly are also important, because bacteria are more likely to thrive on damp skin.

Reduce the risk of bacterial contamination from food

1 Always wash fruits and vegetables thoroughly before peeling or cutting. There have been several cases of gut infection caused by faecal contamination found on produce, believed to be the result of animal or human waste used as fertiliser or someone forgetting to wash their hands after a toilet visit. Be aware that hands are also the main movers of food-poisoning pathogens like *E. coli* and *Salmonella*.

2 Make sure that eggs and meat are cooked properly.

3 Wash hands carefully after handling raw fish, meat and poultry.

4 Avoid eating raw or rare meat and raw fish.

5 Check the recommended temperatures for ice box, freezer and refrigerator, and set yours accordingly.

Be diet wise

Unless you're eating a totally organic diet, assume that a certain percentage of your food intake will inevitably carry some antibiotic residues. These won't be 'wash-offable' so you can't stop them getting into your digestive system. That's why it makes good sense to take regular probiotics and create the right kind of environment in the intestines to help reduce any potential havoc caused by antibiotics in food.

Use herbs and spices

Have you ever pondered on the point that the hotter the climate, and therefore the greater the danger of food going off, the more that spices are used in cooking? Most herbs and spices are naturally antibacterial and many can be considered to have really powerful antibiotic profiles, so it's well worth adding them to some meals. They don't need to be scorchingly strong to make a difference. Why not also make fresh herbs such as parsley, mint, chives, thyme, sage, marjoram and coriander a regular addition to salads and cold dishes? You may be surprised to know that when tested against several different types of bacteria – including *Salmonella* and *Staphylococcus* – garlic, onion, allspice and oregano killed them all, and even the humble chilli pepper was able to dispatch at least 75 per cent of the bad guys. Thyme is strongly antibacterial, as are ginger and turmeric. Not only have some of these herbs and spices been shown to be effective at bumping off the ulcer bug *Helicobacter pylori* but they are also now being used as natural antibacterial additives by the food industry.

Increase the prebiotic content of your diet

There's masses of evidence to show that upping your *prebiotic* intake helps to increase the levels of friendly bacteria in your gut, enabling them to keep pathogenic bacteria under control.

Definitely take probiotics

Thankfully, scientific research has confirmed what many well-informed patients had already worked out for themselves: that probiotics are not only able to relieve the side effects of antibiotics but are also just the ticket when it comes to getting the gut back to normal after antibiotic obliteration. There are several acknowledged experts who think that probiotics should be included as essential post-antibiotic therapy and there's a stack of studies to show that probiotics can be of real benefit in easing the unpleasant symptoms of antibiotic treatment. In particular, one of the most common side effects of antibiotic use – what doctors call AAD (or antibiotic-associated diarrhoea) – responds well to probiotic support (see page 209). Reports also suggest that the intestines of people who take probiotic supplements after antibiotic treatment recolonise more quickly than the intestines of those who don't.

Yet more good reasons, then, why maintaining consistently high levels of friendly flora is such an important part of maintaining human health.

Should you take probiotics at the same time as antibiotics, or afterwards?

It used to be said that there was no point in taking probiotics while on a course of antibiotics, because the drug would kill off the beneficial bacteria in the supplement. Now we have research to support the view that the good gut bugs won't be wasted. Not only do they work hard to reduce the side effects of the antibiotics – especially stomach upset, gas, bloating and erratic bowel movements – but they could also be helping to keep antibiotic-resistant strains at bay and reducing the risk of bad bacteria overgrowing and becoming a problem. Here are some guidelines:

1 When it comes to taking probiotics specifically for the purpose of minimising the effects of antibiotics, research has shown that more is better. So choose products that contain high levels – 20 billion or more – of strains such as *Lactobacillus acidophilus* and *Bifidobacteria*. And get on with it right away. Recolonisation needs

to occur quickly so that the gut gets back to normal, reducing the risk of further infections or the need for yet more antibiotics! After a couple of months or so, everything should be as good as new. However, if you want to continue taking a probiotic supplement after recovery, you could consider reducing the dosage to one that contains, say, between 1 and 10 billion bugs.

2 During the antibiotic course, take the probiotics either immediately before breakfast or an hour or two before bed with a light snack. Most probiotics appreciate a bit of food to help them down. Just remember, whichever time you choose, make sure it's at a different hour of the day to the antibiotic. In other words, don't take your probiotic and antibiotic in the same mouthful; leave not less than three hours between an antibiotic dose and a probiotic dose.

3 Always swallow the probiotic with cold water, never with or near to a hot drink.

When the course of antibiotics is completed, continue the probiotic course for at least another month. If you can afford to do this for longer, say, three months, or even permanently, then so much the better. I would suggest taking the probiotic first thing in the morning, just before breakfast, preferably with a teaspoon or two of milled flaxseed (see page 95).

4 Don't forget that, even if your particular probiotic pack tells you that there is no need for refrigeration (making them very useful if you are travelling and want to take them with you), most probiotic supplements will still be happier being kept in the fridge because it will extend their shelf life.

5 Always check the expiry date before you buy. And don't forget that it will be on your fridge shelf for at least another month after purchase.

6 If the pack doesn't make any mention of how many active live organisms the product contains, then leave it in the shop.

7 Ignore offers that seem like a bargain-hunter's dream. Generally you get what you pay for. In my experience cheap products usually have less effective or non-active ingredients, or are stuffed with unnecessary additives.

8.

Don't Pick Your Nose! The Scary Story of Superbugs

'Human nature forgets unseen foes.'

Sir Alexander Ogston 1844–1929, Scottish surgeon, famous for his
discovery of the bacterium *Staphylococcus aureus*

In years past, posh girls who were pleased about something would use 'super' just as people today say 'cool' or 'great'. So, generally, here is a word we associate with nice things. But there's nothing cool or great about superbugs, which are also known in some countries as superinfections. In this case, the 'super' tag simply stands for a monster with a strength and scope more sinister than perhaps most of us have ever realised.

We know from the previous chapter that antibiotics, as a rule, aren't up to the job anymore, because so many bacteria have developed such clever tactics for ducking and diving their captors. They hide inside cells, swap clothes with each other and adopt aliases to make themselves less easily recognised. But it's worse even than that. Apparently they're also having illicit sex! No, I'm not joking. This isn't just a couple of horny bacteria having it away in a quiet disused cell somewhere. It's the stuff of orgies, a kind of spouse-swapping free-for-all where, instead of exchanging bodily fluids, they trade bits of DNA. Like the expansion of any gene pool, spreading genetic material around strengthens the species, in this case improving the bacteria's resistance to their enemy: the drug that was designed to annihilate them.

Super strains, right from the start

Almost from the moment that antibiotics were born, strains of bacteria were becoming resistant. Rewind to the point where Alexander Fleming was up to his petri dish in penicillin and you'd find the antithesis of his antibiotic already in the making. The very bacterium he was studying when he found the magic mould which started it all had already whistled up a resistant strain. As early as 1946, a mercenary mob of *Staph.* bacteria had found their way into hospital and armed themselves with a new weapon: an enzyme that was able to seek out and destroy the penicillin itself. Scientists fought back with a penicillin upgrade called methicillin, which couldn't be touched by the enzyme armoury. Unfortunately, though, the attacking bugs responded with yet more secretive methods of assault. They used their carnal knowledge of each other to acquire and pass around genetic material, which put a stop to the main function of the new antibiotic; that is, its ability to destroy bacteria by breaking down the cell walls that surround and protect them. The special talent of these clever strains of bacteria lies in their ability to 're-invent' themselves and to spread the resulting resistant strains so that they turn out to be more and more 'anti' towards antibiotics. This particular mutation was named methicillin-resistant *Staphylococcus aureus*, more familiar to us all as MRSA[JB].

How did it come to this?

Staph. bacteria belong to an ancient family of bugs that has been around humans for as long as humans have been around. Home sweet home for *Staph.* is on the skin – always ready to play havoc in open wounds. It's especially happy in dark, damp and warm places – under the arms, in the groin and over the perineum (that wedge of muscle between your genitalia and your anus) – but its favourite haunt is in your hooter. This is why Hugh Pennington, Emeritus Professor of Bacteriology at the University of Aberdeen, and a world-renowned expert on infection and its control, issued his now well-known and incredibly wise words, 'Don't pick your nose.'

MRSA belongs to a family of germs known as *Staphylococcus aureus* and is resistant to a large number of antibiotics, including cephalosporin, penicillin and methicillin, hence its full name: methicillin-resistant *Staphylococcus aureus*.

Symptoms can vary with each patient, but none are nice. First signs of MRSA could be small reddish pimples or boils followed by fever and sometimes a rash. If untreated, the skin eruptions get larger and fill with pus. There may be shivers, low blood pressure, weight loss and raised white cell count. As the disease progresses, there would be widespread infection, damage to vital organs and, in advanced cases, toxic and septic shock or flesh-eating pneumonia.

Treatment may include isolation, drainage of boils, the use of sulphur drugs, antibiotics, strong antibacterial cleansers and antiseptic nose swabs.

Perhaps he might also have added, 'and don't leave the results stuck to surfaces that other people are going to touch'.

Along with a mind-boggling number of its other bacterial buddies, *Staph.* lurks on light switches, trolley handles, escalators, hand rails, doorknobs, lift buttons, desks, computer keyboards and screens, cashpoints, telephones – mobile or otherwise – and almost any other surface you can think of that is stroked, brushed or touched by people.

Are we always in danger?

The good news is that, although we will all probably pick up and carry this germ or one of its close relatives at some time or other throughout our lives, most of us don't even know it. Only when it eyeballs an easy point of entry, such as cuts, grazes or burns, or surgical incisions, does *Staph.* grab its opportunity to invade the body. Even then, if we have good resistance to disease and follow sensible hygiene procedures, the risks are reduced and the immune system will cope. If not, the invader can cause serious infection.

Most common *Staph.* infections start off as abscesses, pressure sores, boils, carbuncles, cellulitis, impetigo, infections of the eyelid, pimples or leg ulcers. More serious cases include blood poisoning, meningitis, or infections that get into the lungs, bone marrow, the lining around the heart or into joints.

When antibiotics first began to be used, most strains of the *Staph.* family would run screaming in terror, give up or die. Infections and illnesses that used to kill people in their hundreds and thousands were being conquered and cured. It was a miracle – but, unfortunately, one that wouldn't last. Having fought back and produced their own weapons to ensure that antibiotics were no longer so effective, the bacteria also began to morph themselves repeatedly into strains that could resist the drugs.

Enter MRSA

The MRSA version of these bacteria is very different to its simple *Staph.* ancestors. For a start, it's far from old; it's taken less than 50 years to work its way from being little more than slightly worrying to becoming a scourge.

The first serious outbreak of MRSA in the 1960s made lots of people very ill but killed only one patient. Statistics change all the time but, as I write this manuscript, officially reported cases of MRSA bloodstream infection are running close to 6,000 a year in the UK with around one in every 500 UK death certificates issued between 2001 and 2005 mentioning MRSA. In the US in 2008, 18,650 people died from the disease. Bear in mind that this includes notified cases only. But it hasn't stopped there. MRSA is clearly intent on going global – an itinerant traveller armed with a case-load of false passports and multiple new identities.

Encouragingly, figures issued by the UK Health Protection Agency show that the numbers of those affected is falling. Unfortunately, however, all superbug statistics are questionable, because there are so many variables to consider; for example, inaccurate diagnoses, some cases not accounted for, others reported incorrectly and, inevitably, mistaken entries on death certificates.

Who is at risk?

Even though it holds the record for becoming the first really famous hospital superbug, the belief that MRSA is confined to hospitals is a myth. It's now found in the community, complete with its own acronym – CA-MRSA (community-associated or community-acquired MRSA). It's most likely to spring up in places where frail or elderly people spend time in close quarters, such as nursing homes or day-care centres, but it is also happy to attack perfectly healthy young people too.

A member of the same family, *Staphylococcus epidermidis*, which is generally harmless until it sees an opportunity to cause trouble, is fond of hitching rides by way of intravenous lines, drainage tubes, catheters, artificial joints or heart valves. It also gets in through body orifices to set up infection in the urinary tract and respiratory system.

How can it be treated?

Treatment for these types of infections is, traditionally, antibiotics – and therein lies the problem. Several newly discovered strains of MRSA are now displaying resistance to even the strongest antibiotics. *Staph. epidermidis* has also changed its appearance, getting stroppy with a number of different antibiotics so that it now has a new name: methicillin-resistant *Staphylococcus epidermidis*: MRSE.

You could be more at risk of picking up MRSA or MRSE if you:

- Are over 65.
- Are very young.
- Have had major surgery.
- Spend a lot of time as a hospital patient or in a long-term convalescent or geriatric-care facility.
- Live in confined circumstances with large groups of other people, such as nursing homes or prisons.
- Have a weakened immune system or a serious long-term illness.
- Are affected by bedsores or leg ulcers.

- Suffer an accidental injury that is not properly treated or protected.
- Play contact sports.
- Bathe, swim or surf in the sea (some coastal waters have been found to have MRSA bacteria).
- Are a pig farmer or a pig. Research shows that the bug is prevalent in both.

Of course, MRSA isn't the only superbug

There's always another superbug waiting in the wings. *Clostridium difficile* (also known as *C. difficile* or *C. diff* for short)[JB] is present in nearly all of us, a natural inhabitant of the gut. If our immune systems are strong and our good gut flora are in charge, it's no problem and is kept well under control. It's when the balance of bacteria in the gut is disrupted for one reason or another that trouble begins to brew; for example, numbers of this bacteria are known to rise following the use of antibiotics.

Clostridium difficile was first identified as a problem in the 1970s and since then, just like MRSA, has become endemic – which means it is constantly present. The UK figures I have at the time of writing show that this infamous bacterium is clocking up around 60,000 reported cases of infection per year with more than 8,000 death certificates mentioning *C. difficile*. It is now considered to be the main cause of hospital-acquired diarrhoea both in Europe and the United States and one of the most common causes of infection of the large intestine.

Where is *C. difficile* found?

Again, like MRSA, we tend to think of *C. difficile* only as a hospital superbug. Put sick, frail or elderly people close together in an area where there is repeated person-to-person contact, add the risk of environmental and surface contamination, multiple use of toilet facilities and difficulties isolating susceptible patients, and *C. difficile* thinks it's Christmas! But it can attack anywhere and, along with MRSA, has now spread from the cosy confines of hospital wards out into the community.

Clostridium difficile is the name we give to the actual bacterium, but the condition that it causes is known as *Clostridium difficile* colitis. Once the infection has taken hold, toxins are produced that create symptoms of abdominal pain, fever, vomiting, elevated white cell count, severe inflammation of the colon and urgent diarrhoea with consequent dehydration. In serious cases the disease can progress to something called pseudomembraneous colitis (PMC), which damages the lining of the gut, perforating the colon wall and allowing the infection to leak into the abdomen, often with life-threatening results. This is why anyone who has recently been in hospital and been pre-scribed antibiotics in the past three months and who then develops diarrhoea and pain, should seek urgent medical advice.

The name *Clostridium* derives from a Greek word meaning 'spindle' (which describes the shape of the bacterium). And the word *difficile* means 'difficult'. It is, literally, a difficult spindle to get rid of; in bacterial terms: a tough cookie that's hard to control and impossible to completely eradicate.

Hospital treatment of *C. difficile*-related colitis usually includes more antibiotics, fluids to rehydrate the system, drugs to target the toxins, and, in an ideal world, isolation from other patients until the crisis has passed.

As a rule, here is a bug that prefers to take advantage where someone has had antibiotics. (Because these drugs upset the normal balance of bacteria in the large bowel, it's easier for *C. difficile* to set up home there.) The more courses of antibiotics, the greater the risk. But there's another problem. Although less likely, it's possible to pick up a *C. difficile* infection without having taken antibiotics in the recent past. So, to be in the loop, not only do you *not* have to be a hospital patient, you don't necessarily need to have been prescribed antibiotics either. No one can yet be sure why this is, but it seems perfectly possible that the bacteria could be on the lookout for anyone who has poor levels of good gut bacteria and therefore less protection.

You're more at risk if you:

- Have had antibiotics in the past 45–90 days.
- Are over 65.
- Have had any kind of surgery.
- Are taking any kind of regular drug that suppresses stomach acid (see page 135).
- Already have some type of gastrointestinal disease, such as Crohn's, ulcerative colitis or irritable bowel syndrome.
- Suffer from any kind of immune-system disorder.
- Have no spleen.
- Are undergoing chemotherapy.
- Have a weak chest.
- Have poor resistance to illness for some other reason.
- Are a long-term inpatient or a resident in a nursing home.
- Have a disturbed balance of gut bacteria.

Transmission and reinfection are easy-peasy

There's a busy traffic of C. *difficile* to and fro between communities and hospitals. What often happens is that a person contracts the infection while in hospital, but the diarrhoea symptoms don't manifest themselves until they're discharged, maybe to their own home or perhaps to convalescent or residential care. When the illness is discovered, they're then almost certainly going to need serious medical support. But, by this time, it's likely that the bug has already spread to other people and will also probably bounce back to the same or another hospital, ready and willing to attack yet another weak and unsuspecting individual. Something else we all need to be aware of is that it's possible to contract the infection and have no symptoms at all, yet still be a carrier who is able to pass the bacteria on to someone else.

Not only is C. *difficile* demonstrating resistance to antibiotics but it has also developed other clever ways to survive. There is concern that strong antibacterial cleaners may no longer be up to the task of killing it. And while heat, certainly above 80°C (176°F), is death to most bacteria, some members of the effluent-loving *Clostridia* family are frustratingly resistant to high temperatures; for example, where the vast majority of microbes will keel over quite quickly in a hot pan, certain types of *Clostridia* have survived long hours of boiling and even steam at 120°C (248°F).

One thing they don't like is acidity. It's already known that strong solutions of vinegar and hot water may turn out to be at least as effective, if not more so, than regular cleaning fluids for killing a variety of different bacteria on surfaces. This may also be one reason at least why consuming foods and supplements containing lactic acid bacteria helps to improve our resistance.

New members of the Antibiotic Resistance Movement

I've highlighted MRSA and *C. difficile* because these two are the best-known superbugs. But they're not the only ones, nor the worst.

Today, we're faced with a whole array of other resistant bacteria and related illnesses that are becoming more and more difficult to remedy, most with unfamiliar and often hard-to-pronounce names such as *Pseudomonas aeruginosa*, which hangs about on hospital equipment such as respirators, catheters and tubing, and *Stenotrophomonas maltophilia*, which makes moist places its home and is happy in showers, showerheads, taps, sinks and plugs.

Then there's *Streptococcus pneumoniae*, implicated in meningitis, septicaemia and, as its name suggests, 'classical' pneumonia. And *Enterococcus*, a bacterium that can cause urinary, blood and skin infections, and has now become resistant to the strongest of antibiotics. It's also modified itself to withstand all but the most vigorous levels of hygiene and can lie in wait on cracked, pitted, unclean or badly cleaned surfaces for months. *E. coli*, although famous for food-poisoning outbreaks, is a normal gut dweller and usually causes no problems in healthy people. Now, pathogenic *E. coli* not only resists antibiotics but has also mutated and, again just like MRSA, has armed itself with an enzyme gun so that it can zap the drugs and make them useless. *Klebsiella* is another bug that cohabits with humans and generally caused few problems in those with strong immunity. Now it, too, has joined the Antibiotic Resistance Movement, working undercover to cause havoc in hospitals, with special responsibility for kidney, lung and blood infections, and likes nothing more than sneaking under its invisibility cloak and finding its way into intensive-care and neo-natal units.

Bugs hitch rides on anything that moves

Bacteria love to travel and will go where people go. Baby buggies (perhaps well named), supermarket trolleys and medicine trolleys, as well as mobile cleaning units that are pushed around hospital wards and in and out of public washrooms, can all spread bacteria around. So, too, can the undersides of briefcases, handbags, carrier bags and shoppers that we dump on the floor when we visit the ladies – or gents. Then, unwittingly, we give those same bacteria a free ride home and unload them on the kitchen worktop.

That's only the half of it. Stomach upsets, food poisoning, diarrhoea, throat infections, poor wound healing – the risk of all these things would be less, say experts, if we paid more attention to basic hygiene.

Getting hygiene right

Transmission of bacteria from visitors and staff to patients, and vice versa, is a huge problem that is still not being addressed in all hospitals. Staff who don't stick to set-down sanitary procedures can very easily transfer bacteria between wards and from patient to patient. And it's even easier for visitors to spread bugs to or from toilets, into the cafeteria, down in the lift and then outside the building. Toilet seats are a big risk area for *C. difficile* because it takes only the tiniest touch of a contaminated finger or a splash of infected diarrhoea waste to ensure transfer to another person.

Seek, isolate and destroy

Much of the time, thank goodness, our immune systems clock any bacteria that look as if they might be about to cause illness. Our internal police force won't necessarily obliterate them all, but it can keep them under control. Trouble comes when immunity is low or the bad bugs have taken a particularly strong hold. That's when eradicating superbugs becomes hard work. First you have to find them, then segregate them and, if you're lucky, wipe them out. Isolating the sufferers and stuffing them full of the strongest available antibiotics isn't the only answer and doesn't always work. Stringent barrier nursing is known to be essential and yet, in many places, not even the simplest precautions are being followed. Scrupulous hygiene is vital. *Clostridium difficile*, MRSA, and their dangerous friends, are opportunists that spread by contact from surface to surface and person to person and, as a result, are more likely to be rampant where cleanliness is found wanting.

Taking a backward glance for treatment?

Clever people are continually coming up with new ideas. One is an innovative approach known as phage therapy (short for bacteriophage), a type of virus that attacks bacteria such as MRSA. Another is a gel that destroys the bacteria in the nose. Treatment of *C. difficile* with a yeast known as *Saccharomyces boulardii* has been shown to relieve symptoms and encourage healing, perhaps because the yeast is able to destroy the toxin. In another study, *C. difficile* infections were reduced significantly by the use of some of our familiar probiotic pals *Lactobacillus bulgaricus*, *L. acidophilus* and *Bifidobacteria*.

Inevitably, new kinds of antibiotics are coming on-stream but who knows how long it will be before the bacteria have stolen another march on medical technology. Scientists are trying to beat them back by using nanotechnology to isolate which new drugs will do the trick.

In the end, it may be Mother Nature who comes to our rescue. If we needed proof that sometimes the old ways are the best, have a look at these:

- *Pulsatilla vulgaris* (pasque flower) and *Inula helenium* (elecampane), which are already highly prized as medicinal herbs, have turned out to have formidable bug-bashing abilities. When extracts from both these wild flowers were pitted against a wide range of *Staph.* bacteria, the pasque flower plant was found to be extremely effective against MRSA and the elecampane annihilated 100 per cent of this persistent superbug.

- Research also confirms that plants, including tea tree, manuka, oregano, geranium and melissa, contain essential oils that have strong antibacterial qualities, and that natural herbals such as basil, blueberry, elderberry, echinacea, geranium-seed extract, olive leaf and St John's Wort are justifiably prized for their bacteria-beating ability.

- Raw garlic is an age-old fighter of bacterial infection that has now been 're-discovered' as an effective MRSA missile.

- And, although we might not care to think about it too closely, maggot therapy has been used recently and successfully in hospital to destroy the MRSA in diabetic ulcers.

How about a poo implant?

Although the thought of it might sound disgusting, did you know that one person's poo could be the source of another person's recovery? Implanted sections of stool taken from a healthy person and inserted into the intestines of those with severe bacterial imbalance have been shown to help patients recover from *Clostridium difficile* colitis. Experts believe the reason for the success is because the stool from the healthy volunteer rectifies the imbalance by repopulating the gut with billions of beneficial bacteria.

More common-sense solutions

If we're to make any speedy inroads into this extremely scary superbug situation, it may be that the most important remedies are in our own (clean) hands.

- If you have a history of taking antacid or anti-ulcer medication (their use and overuse is incredibly common), then make sure you are regularly reviewed by your GP. If you're not sure, check your prescription with a pharmacist or look it up on the Internet. Long-term intake of drugs known as H2 receptor antagonists and proton pump inhibitors are linked to an increased risk of *C. difficile*-associated infection, especially in the elderly. It's suspected that any drugs that suppress gastric acid allow the bacteria to proliferate, because the stomach is too alkaline to kill them off. Such medicines also have a range of other hidden side effects and, while valuable in the short-term, are not supposed to be taken over an extended period of time. Even the pharmaceutical companies who make them recommend that acid-suppressors are used for short-term treatment only. If you're treating yourself with over-the-counter medicines because you have discomfort that feels like indigestion, it's also worth getting a check-up. Many a heart problem has been mistaken for acidity, and vice versa.

- Many elderly people already suffer with naturally low levels of stomach acid (hypochlorhydria) brought on by ageing, and so will be at similar risk. There is already evidence that achlorhydria (complete lack of stomach acid) can result in bacterial overgrowth in the small intestine – a condition known as SIBO (see page 214). If you're suffering problems with acidity, gastro-oesophageal reflux disease (GORD) or hiatus hernia, then these medicines used in the short term can be helpful, but there are several other routes you might try before resorting to permanent medication. My experience as a practitioner has proved many times over that looking more closely into a patient's eating habits and making adjustments to diet can be incredibly helpful. Sad, then, that nutritional therapy is so rarely considered a priority and, especially in the UK, often dismissed as a last resort.

- Take common-sense hygiene precautions against hazardous bacteria. The most effective antibacterial safeguard is to wash our hands, preferably several times a day and always in hot soapy water. There are quite a few natural products now available which are effective without using harsh chemicals. See Chapter 7 and Resources.

- Don't use someone else's towel, facecloth or toothbrush, or share clothing that hasn't been washed in between times.

- If you cut, graze or scald yourself, clean and cover any wounds with a plaster or bandage to prevent them becoming contaminated or infected. The same applies if you sustain a skin injury on the sports field. There are several reports of young people succumbing to superbug infections as a result of apparently simple sports injuries. If you have a skin problem that won't heal, see your doctor immediately. Remember an open wound, however small, is the most common route into the body for *Staph.* bacteria. Use a natural antibacterial soap in the shower and wash towels and sports gear after every use. Don't walk barefoot in the locker room or gym.

- Essential oils make excellent antibacterial skin cleansers when added to water for bathing or washing the face and hands. Choose a pH-balanced liquid handwash and add a few drops of pure oil to each new bottle to enhance its bug-killing qualities. Cinnamon oil, melissa, oregano, lemongrass, lemon myrtle, mountain savory, neem oil, manuka and tea tree oil all have an antibacterial punch and some have been shown in laboratory studies to inhibit the growth of MRSA. See box below.

Take care
Here are a few important cautions when using essential oils:
- Always use the best-quality essential oils and beware of cheap products; those that seem like a bargain may be missing the vital active ingredients.
- Follow the pack instructions carefully.
- Use sparingly; a very small quantity is all that's required.
- Never apply essential oils directly to the skin; always dilute them first into water or a carrier oil.
- Never take them internally.

- Pure aloe vera is well known as an excellent treatment for minor burns (including sunburn) but also works well for pressure sores and other skin abrasions. Products that claim to be aloe based but show it right at the bottom of the list of ingredients may contain too small an amount to have any useful benefit. I have used Aloe 99 from Xynergy Health Products for many years, because it's so pure and so effective. Also really helpful is High Strength Comvita Manuka Honey (which you can take internally as well as using to dress infections) and Organix Neem Leaf & Aloe Gel. Both available from selected health stores and direct from www.xynergy.co.uk.

- Get support from your diet. Eat foods that are rich in antioxidant vitamins A, C and E, selenium and zinc. Include plenty of fresh vegetables, salad foods, fruit and fruit juices. They can be truly valuable defences in the battle against infection. Take a daily serving of a probiotic drink or live yoghurt, buttermilk or kefir. Add garlic to your menus.

- Remind yourself of the care advice in Chapter 7 (page 114).

Care as an inpatient

If you have to go to hospital as an inpatient, here are some things to help protect you from infections:

- Insist that nurses and doctors wash their hands before touching or examining you. Someone who was recently in hospital told me that she saw doctors and nurses going from one bed to another without any use of disinfectant, hot water or change of gloves in between. The ward next to hers was an isolation area for a patient with *C. difficile*, but the door was left permanently open. The same medicine and cleaning trolleys were wheeled into the infected room and then out into the normal ward without any interim swabbing. Even magazines and newspapers were exchanged between this and other wards!

- If the toilets aren't clean, make a fuss or get a visitor or relative to complain on your behalf. If nothing happens, ask to be transferred.

- If any of the doctors or consultants is wearing a tie or unbuttoned jacket or white coat that's flapping around, don't let them dangle the fabric over you when they're carrying out any examination or treatment. There's a concern that medics' wild and unrestrained clothing might pick up bacteria from other patients and pass them around. MRSA is known to survive long term on fabrics, including privacy curtains, bedcovers and overalls.

- Take a bottle of tea tree essential oil with you and, if you can't do it yourself, get someone to put a few drops into a bowl of hot water and use it to wipe down your locker and wash the floor around the bed as often as is possible. In Russia, by the way, they put raw garlic in the cleaning water. It's a cheap and very effective antibacterial.

- Keep your nose clean. Use disposable tissues, not cotton handkerchiefs. If you're keen on reducing the risk of infection and need to clean your nostrils, use antiseptic wet-wipes and, if you need to blow, wash hands thoroughly afterwards. The nose is such a good place for *Staph.* bacteria to hide that it's not uncommon for hospitals to take nose swabs to screen for MRSA. Some medics recommend, every day for the first week at home, to very gently swab the nostrils using cotton buds and then to apply mupirocin (Bactroban) ointment and to encourage anyone else in the house to do the same. Remember: the bacteria responsible for MRSA infection loves the inside of your nose.

- I'm sure you already know that there are protection packs now available that contain cleansing wipes, hand-sanitising spray, hair and body wash and fabric spray. Anyone who suggests that these things are not necessary has probably never been an inpatient in an at-risk hospital. One place to be exceedingly generous in your use of disinfectant wipes is the toilet seat, where *C. difficile* can very easily be deposited from another patient. Offer antiseptic hand wipes to all visitors, including medical personnel if you have the slightest doubt that they may not have washed their hands. Your life may depend upon it.

- Once discharged, continue to use antibacterial soap for head-to-toe bathing or showering for at least a week or until full recovery. If, like me, you prefer to avoid unnecessary chemical ingredients, check out organic suppliers, independent health stores and online sellers who use natural ingredients. I've included some of them in Resources. Something else I often do is to buy a plain organic liquid soap from the health store and add a few drops of one of my favourite antibacterial oils, such as Thursday Plantation Tea Tree Oil, Bioforce Neem Oil or Comvita Manuka Oil. When someone is convalescing, it's also nice (and an additional bug deterrent) to add essential oils to a diffuser in the room.

> **Take care**
> If you're visiting anyone in hospital who is in one of the risk groups mentioned in this chapter, wear gloves, especially if you're helping with their bathing or other nursing tasks. Ask for a protective apron and wash your hands before and after seeing the patient.

Protect your insides, too

However good the external cleansing of the surfaces around you, you still need help to boost your internal immunity. This is why I would very highly recommended the following:

- If you have an operation or some hospital treatment or test pending, try to start probiotics at least a week before you're admitted. If possible, continue to take them during your stay (with the agreement of your doctor), even if it's only a day procedure, and for at least 60 days after you return home. Do this whether you're taking antibiotics or not.

- Buy Dr Vogel's Echinaforce. This is even more important if you belong to any of the at-risk groups on page 127 or 130. I've seen echinacea produce many incredible results. I recommend it to all my patients. Echinaforce, a registered medicine, is proven to help reduce the duration of cold symptoms, but I've also found it to be extremely effective at boosting the immune system and dealing with other infections too. Take 20 drops twice daily for a week before you go into hospital, carry on using it all through your stay (except when you're 'nil by mouth'), and continue for a month after you're discharged. Obviously, you will need to tell the hospital that you are taking this herbal medicine but, in my experience, there's usually no objection. Recently, as I write, a colleague of mine was admitted for a major heart operation. He followed the above advice and took probiotics every day, and he was the *only* person in a unit of 16 people who did *not* go down with a post-op infection.

- In addition to the Echinaforce, I like to keep my first-aid cabinet stocked with Bionutri's Elderberry Complex and also Comvita Olive Leaf Complex in case extra backup is needed during an infection.

A tip too far?

If you're inclined to think that all this information is a bit over the top, consider the consequences of not protecting ourselves. Apart from the inconvenience, the pain and the suffering, there is a massive risk of passing these life-threatening infections on to other people. The cost to the NHS and other health-care providers of caring for and treating sufferers is incalculable, not only in terms of time and resources but in money, too. Prevention costs peanuts compared to the thousands of pounds spent on supporting sick and vulnerable patients who might not have contracted the illness in the first place if only more precautions had been taken.

Before the advent of antibiotics, people died in their thousands from bacterial illness. For a brief blip in our modern medical history, death rates from all kinds of infectious diseases were dramatically decreased and many lives were saved by these miracle medicines. Now, though, as pathogenic bacteria evolve constantly in order to beat the system, infectious diseases are once again becoming untreatable or non-responsive. It's easy to be depressed that we've come full circle, but let's be grateful that, thanks to continued research, we also have so much more knowledge and new information about how best to protect ourselves.

9.

If You Do Nothing Else . . .

‘Your time is limited, so don't waste it living someone else's life. Don't be trapped by dogma – which is living with the results of other people's thinking. Don't let the noise of other's opinions drown out your own inner voice. And most important, have the courage to follow your heart and intuition.’

Steve Jobs, Co-founder of Apple

I know I've already given you a lot of information to take on board. And although not everything will apply to you, I'm guessing that a great chunk of it probably will. But I'm also very much aware that it's unlikely you'll get around to using all that you need. You're not the only one. I'm just as guilty. The difference is that I take special care of my diet and never eat rubbish food. I breathe deeply, chew thoroughly and generally practise what I preach. That's not because I'm a goody two-shoes, it's just that I know how much extra strength and coping power I get by following these simple health-boosting recommendations, even though modern life is busy.

However much anyone wants to get well, it often seems that there is simply no breathing space to make the changes – too much else gets in the way. You don't need me to tell you how important it is for you to be a priority in your own life, to stop putting everything else and everyone else first and to take care of yourself. Don't let life's stresses and strains swamp all your best intentions. Please don't wait until something serious is diagnosed before you take charge.

I've added this section for those who know they need to take some action now but are unlikely to get through all the relevant chapters in this book. There are 20 top tips here, all aimed at giving your diet a quick makeover which, even at this level, will help not only to support your good gut bugs but also to make you feel much better. If you do nothing else, read them through and then promise yourself that you'll introduce them, one or two at a time, into your daily routine. When you begin to pick up, perhaps you'll feel like diving in more detail into other chapters.

Emergency action plan

Here are my 20 top tips for breathing, posture, diet and general healthy living:

1 Breathe more deeply and more slowly. Check yourself, especially if you are rushed or stressed. When did you last take a deep breath?

2 Check your posture. Open up that cramped chest and relax your shoulders. Did you realise that you don't breathe properly if you are crouched or tense, which means that you won't digest properly either? It's common to see people lean right over their meal as if they were worried someone was going to steal it. If you can, sit relaxed but straight, so that your stomach and belly aren't rolled up together in front of you. It's why dining chairs are better for your posture and your digestion than either eating standing up or slumping in front of the television. Posture also applies to computer keyboards; don't lean forward over the desk while you're typing or using the mouse.

3 Eat at the table. Try to avoid eating meals in front of the TV. You may not think it's stressing your digestion, but television programmes are designed to stimulate and they won't be good for your gut in any way at all.

4 Chew your food. Give your digestion and your bowel function a real helping hand by masticating each mouthful thoroughly before swallowing. This can help the 'terrain' inside your intestines and make the internal environment better for your good gut bugs. Try pausing and resting the eating irons between mouthfuls. Do you have an urgent appointment? Will the world be under threat if you slow down? It's much better to take your time and savour the taste of the food than behave as if you were in a competition to see who can finish first.

5 Respect your digestion and give it all the help you can; for example, try to eat regular meals. If that's not possible, at least have access to healthy snacks throughout the day. It's a big mistake to run on empty from the minute you get up in the morning, to skip lunch and then fill up on a big meal in the evening. And never eat on the move. Always stop and sit down to eat. It's vital for good gut health and for encouraging good gut bugs to thrive.

6 Drink more fluid. If you find this difficult, here's a way of increasing the volume without realising it. Leave 2 litre ($3^1/_2$ pint) bottles of water somewhere where you spend most of your day, and drink from them regularly. It's a good way to check how much you get through in 24 hours. You can either refill these from a filter jug or buy bottled water. I prefer to avoid the chlorine and risk of antibiotic or other chemical residues in tap water. Put one or more glasses, or bottles, on your desk or in the bathroom or kitchen – wherever you're most likely to see them and take mouthfuls throughout the day. If you're on the move, carry smaller bottles of water with you in the car or in your bag. Drink a full glass of water every morning when you first get up and take another full glass with every meal.

7 Eat the right kind of dietary fibre (including the addition of flaxseed on a daily basis – see below). See Chapter 2 and page 85 on prebiotics. This is one of the most important things you can do for your health, and your good gut bugs will love you for it.

8 Take flaxseed every day. Try two teaspoons of flaxseed with a glass of water every morning before breakfast. You can put it onto breakfast cereal or take it with yoghurt, but if you do this, it's really important that you also have a full glass of water as well. If flax isn't available or not to your taste, psyllium husk fibre is also excellent.

And always remember this: fibre needs fluid to work properly (see page 99).

9 Get those bowels moving. Read the very important notes in Chapter 2, page 41, and also page 202 of Chapter 16.

10 Be honest about your alcohol intake. Make certain that you know what a unit of wine, beer or spirits actually looks like. Page 44 has useful interactive websites so that you can check your intake. When you do drink, remember that alcohol doesn't contribute to your daily fluid intake, so it helps to take a glass of water for each glass of alcohol.

11 Do whatever you can to avoid smoking. If you're a determined smoker who just won't quit or has given up trying, at least consider that your smoke could be affecting someone else's health. For sure, it will be affecting yours, so give your body the best protection you can by increasing your intake of nutrient-rich vegetables and fruit.

12 Aim for that all-important five-a-day target. I know there's that not-so-old saying that we'd all live longer if green vegetables smelled as good as bacon. But even though they don't, there are lots of really delicious ways of prepping veg to make it really appetising. If you find vegetables revolting it's probably because they've been boiled to death in big pieces in too much water. Waterless cooking, steaming or sautéing, is healthier and retains more flavour. Chopping vegetables (and salad foods) into smaller pieces makes them much more attractive. If your lot hate greens, make a purée by blending cooked vegetables, and add to sauces or gravies. Fry an onion and stir it into mashed broccoli, cabbage or sprouts. Use a little butter and salt if it helps get them down. Neither will kill you and you'll need only small amounts. Cook carrots by adding a little olive oil and 'steaming' them on the lowest heat with the lid clamped on tightly. Shake them occasionally to prevent sticking. The result is tender and succulent.

There are lots of other ways of upping that five-a-day: how about a piece of fruit before breakfast? Eat dried fruit such as dates, apricots, figs, sultanas and raisins on your breakfast cereal. Have another piece of fresh fruit, or maybe a small fruit salad, as a starter before lunch or evening meal. Enjoy a glass of fresh fruit juice (with pulp) or a fruit smoothie instead of coffee. Add salad to that sandwich or as an extra side dish. Include two fresh vegetables (other than potatoes or peas) with your main meal of the day. And remember, it's easy to 'hide' extra servings of vegetables in stir-fries, stews and casseroles, and to blend them into soups.

13 Wash all fresh produce thoroughly before use to remove surface chemical residues.

14 Do without the sump oil. It's long been my view that nobody needs margarine-type spreads or foods that contain the 'H' word (H for hydrogenated fats and oils). I believe that it's an excess of these wrong types of fat that contribute to elevated cholesterol and cardiovascular problems. Try as I might, I can find no evidence anywhere that butter is the cause of heart disease. If you need a spread, then a scraping of unsalted butter has to be a better option than heavily processed oil. Or, better still, why not use things like hummus or ripe avocado pear as a spread? Both are incredibly healthy foods.

15 Use the Swap Box that begins on page 50 and introduce as many of the recommendations as you can into your regular daily routine.

16 Try to eat less of those foods that are not kind to the gut, especially fry-ups, pizzas, burgers, red meat – particularly pork and sliced meats (they usually contain preservatives) – packaged ready meals, sugar and sugary foods, cakes, biscuits and desserts that are high in fat or sugar, or contain artificial sweeteners.

17 Become an avid label reader. Check packaging every time you buy a food item and be horrified at how many E numbers, stabilisers, emulsifiers, flavours, colours, preservatives, bulking agents and other chemical-sounding names so many products contain. Be aware that so much of what's on the supermarket shelves is loaded with salt, sugar or chemical sweeteners. Sometimes, it's a wonder that there's enough room left for the food itself. It's only when you realise how much junk there really is in junk food that you might think about looking around for healthier alternatives.

18 Don't let your body become a storage container for pseudo-foods. Be aware that anything trumpeting that it's low in calories or has zero fat is almost always going to be weighing heavy with manufactured mush to replace the fat, sugar or whatever else has been removed. It might not be the good deal you were promised, and chances are that you'll be paying a higher price for it in more ways than one.

19 Read Chapter 4 on prebiotic foods and try to incorporate some of the recommendations into your diet.

20 Make probiotics a regular part of your diet. Eat at least one, preferably two servings of fermented-milk products (yoghurt, probiotic shots, kefir, buttermilk) every day. Invest regularly in the best-quality probiotic supplement you can afford. Take it year round if you can, but if not, at least follow a two- or three-month course with top-ups as and when you can afford them and *always* after antibiotics. I take my probiotic supplement along with my flaxseed and water before breakfast. As far as I'm concerned, it's simply good health insurance.

Part Two

Probiotic Support for Particular Problems

10.

How Disease Begins in the Gut: Dealing with Dysbiosis

Dysbiosis is a term that was coined specifically to describe an imbalance of bacteria in the gut – and it's a real Nasty Nigel. Why? Because it can compromise the immune system and is a major player in many different diseases. When we put dys- or dis- in front of any word it indicates something is wrong, ill, bad or abnormal, as in dysfunction, distress, disturbance, disharmony or disease. Hence dysbiosis.

Suspect dysbiosis if you suffer regularly with symptoms such as constipation, diarrhoea, bloating, wind or cystitis. It can also be a factor in joint pain, headaches, insomnia and fatigue. If left untreated, some practitioners believe it could contribute to more serious conditions such as chronic fatigue syndrome (ME), inflammatory bowel diseases such as Crohn's disease and ulcerative colitis, irritable bowel syndrome (IBS), ankylosing spondylitis, rheumatoid arthritis, multiple sclerosis and a condition known as leaky gut syndrome.

Dysbiosis may also be a factor for people suffering allergies, eczema and psoriasis, in hormonal disturbance and in seemingly unrelated emotional problems that can cause mood changes, anxiety and depression. Although it's certainly not a symptomless condition, it's often the case that people are unaware that their health is being compromised by this type of imbalance.

Welcome to the dysbiotic dumping ground

When balance is maintained, the various colonies of bacteria that share our body space are beneficial to us. They all have a specific purpose and do us no harm. In fact, they're actually necessary for our survival. That's what symbiosis is all about. Not only do the different types of bacteria protect the body, each community of different microbes works together and keeps an eye on each other to make sure that no particular group gets smart-alecky and tries to take over.

But where there's dysbiosis, this democratic system breaks down so that one unwanted colony might get bigger while another that we need might be seriously damaged or disappear altogether. This scenario could be repeated many times over so that, in the end, the whole ecology of the gut is completely upset.

Worse still, when dysbiosis is in full swing and bacterial colonies are not functioning properly, there's the added problem of what to do with the garbage. Toxic waste isn't confined to the problems of landfill sites, factory fall-out or polluted rivers. It's going on inside the body too. The microorganisms that we've been talking about here all have to get rid of their own rubbish; just as we have to empty our bowels every day and our refuse bins every week. The wastes themselves begin to putrefy and produce their own noxious gases; pockets and crevices in the colon get choked with decomposing excreta and all the while more poo is being piled on top of the heap. Not surprisingly, bad bacteria love this kind of environment. As far as they're concerned, the more disgusting, the better. No wonder a dysbiotic gut rumbles and farts so much when it becomes dysfunctional and disturbed.

What are the causes of dysbiosis?

It seems likely that one of the main triggers could be the repeated use of medicines such as antibiotics, anti-ulcer drugs and steroids. Poor-quality diet is also a big issue, especially if it lacks variety, is heavy on meat, low on vegetables, lacking in prebiotic foods (see Chapter 4) and hasn't enough good-quality fibre; or if it relies too much on packaged processed foods and is high in sugar and/or chemical additives.

And then there's the environmental impact of pollution on the system and yet more chemicals from household cleaning products and agrichemicals. You'd be surprised how easy it is to turn your body into chemical city.

The chemical connection

If you don't have a garden and don't have fields nearby, you may think that you're not likely to be exposed to herbicides, insecticides, fungicides or pesticides. But be aware. These chemicals, designed to kill insect pests, bacteria, viruses and fungi on the plant, are routinely sprayed onto the crops that become the grains, fruits and vegetables you eat. It doesn't necessarily mean those 'Farmaceuticals' have stopped working once the crop has been harvested. They can affect you and your intestines, too. You might be reassured by manufacturer statements that agrichemicals are classed as safe for use but, unfortunately, your body isn't all that impressed and would really rather you steered clear of them. Your system already receives a daily onslaught of 'multi' chemicals around the home, including cleaning fluids, skincare, hair and shower products, toothpaste, the gases given off by carpets, plastics and polystyrene, air fresheners, loo blocks ... the list is endless.

Auto-intoxication

In almost every case of dysbiosis, there will be yet another problem brewing and that's an overgrowth of yeast fungus. And what does yeast love best? Sugar, of course. All we have to do to make a bad situation much worse is to fuel the body with a diet that's high in sugar, sugary foods and alcohol. The yeasts shout 'whoopee' and get completely paralytic with power, hooking themselves onto the gut wall, damaging the permeable membrane between the gut and the bloodstream and causing leaky gut syndrome, and possibly also laying the groundwork for a condition known as candidiasis (see page 246).

It just gets worse

By the time we get to this stage, we probably start reacting to foods that never used to be a problem. The immune system is on full alert. Now we have allergies to add to the load. Because of the allergies and the yeasts and the damage to the gut wall, we aren't digesting properly anymore. The body is no longer able to absorb the nourishment provided by our food supply. The immune system, already overworked, isn't getting the nutrients it needs to fight off the invaders. If we weren't breastfed as a baby, this will also, almost certainly, affect conditions in the gut in later life.

Antibiotics

Of course, antibiotics are designed to eradicate unwanted bacteria. Sometimes they work and sometimes they don't. The downside, as we've seen in Chapter 7, is that they also wipe out beneficial gut flora at the same time. The more courses of antibiotics someone takes, generally the higher the risk of dysbiosis occurring. With this constant wipe-out of good gut bugs leaving the intestines unprotected, pathogenic bacteria get their nasty little feet back under the table very quickly and invite all their dangerous and disgusting yeasty and wormy friends to join them. Drunk on power and deaf to all reasoning, they get together and release a whole range of poisonous chemicals and toxic substances into the gut and the bloodstream, including ammonia, hydrogen sulphide (which causes that niffy smell of rotten eggs), and other stuff you don't really want to know about, including secondary bile acids, amines and phenols; no wonder then that when the normally harmonious colony of gut microbes becomes unbalanced or destroyed in this way, chronic ill health can be the result. And it's not just the gut that is upset. Almost any internal or external skin surface can be affected; for example, oral dysbiosis (in the mouth) or vaginal dysbiosis.

There have been many wise and experienced doctors of what I would call 'the old school' who believe that a range of health problems are likely to be caused by a dysbiotic (toxic) gut, poor diet and the overuse of pharmaceutical medicines. Currently, however,

From digestive distress to dysbiosis and disease

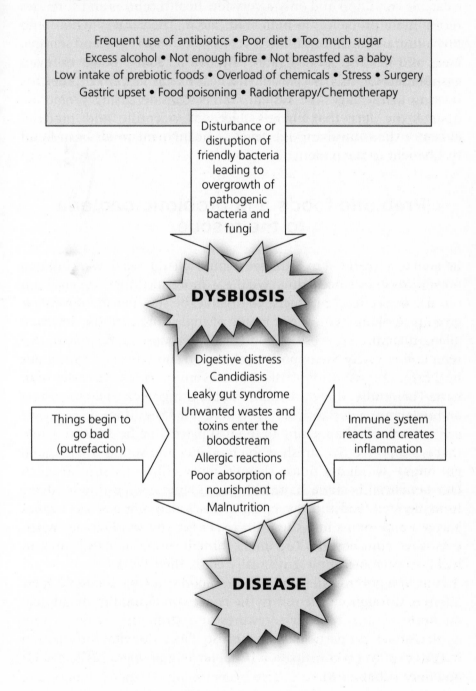

Frequent use of antibiotics • Poor diet • Too much sugar
Excess alcohol • Not enough fibre • Not breastfed as a baby
Low intake of prebiotic foods • Overload of chemicals • Stress • Surgery
Gastric upset • Food poisoning • Radiotherapy/Chemotherapy

Disturbance or disruption of friendly bacteria leading to overgrowth of pathogenic bacteria and fungi

DYSBIOSIS

Things begin to go bad (putrefaction)

Digestive distress
Candidiasis
Leaky gut syndrome
Unwanted wastes and toxins enter the bloodstream
Allergic reactions
Poor absorption of nourishment
Malnutrition

Immune system reacts and creates inflammation

DISEASE

the medical profession generally doesn't recognise dysbiosis as a treatable condition and only a very few health centres and surgeries recommend probiotics to help eradicate it. The surgery where I do my voluntary nutrition clinics is very open to these safe and sensible ideas and has the success rates to prove it. Sadly, however, even gastroenterologists (specialists who deal exclusively with problems relating to the digestive system) rarely consider using probiotics, despite the fact that there's excellent scientific and practical evidence that improving the level of healthy microflora can be of real benefit to the patient.

Prebiotic foods and probiotic bacteria to the rescue

In an ideal world, I'm sure we would all do what we could to prevent dysbiosis occurring. We'd eat more healthily, cut back on our use of chemical products, go organic, be sensible about alcohol, give up smoking, reduce our intake of sugar, and read the labels on all manufactured processed foods! Well, perhaps. Sadly, though, we tend to do exactly the opposite, relying on shortcuts and taking our health for granted until it fails. But prevention is always easier than cure. Thankfully, there are many simple things we can do to correct and rebalance a dysbiotic gut, and it's even easier if we do what we can to prevent it happening in the first place. In a healthy gut – one that is supported by a fresh wholefood diet and supplied with good gut bugs – we find a much cleaner, more efficiently run business. Our beneficial bacteria have a delicious time composting leftovers from digested foodstuff, sweeping up discarded cells and kicking old bacteria and toxins into the trash ready for you to move out when you move your bowels! You might think it sounds like the job from hell but, trust me, these guys really enjoy their work.

Your first port of call should be the Good Gut Upgrade in Chapter 2. Then, throughout the rest of the book, you'll find first-hand help on how to nurture your intestines and strengthen your system against attack. In particular, please also check the vital information in the chapters on constipation (Chapter 16), prebiotics (Chapter 4) and fibre (Chapter 6).

At the very least make sure you read Chapter 9.

11.

Good Gut Bugs and Allergies

Research confirms that allergic reactions – and associated inflammation – are more likely where good gut microbes are in short supply. Or put another way, people who suffer with allergies generally have lower levels of healthy gut flora. There are several studies ongoing in different parts of the world to see if taking probiotics might make a difference to the lives of asthma and allergy sufferers, in particular by switching off the inflammatory responses that are caused when the immune system overreacts.

If you're plagued by respiratory allergies, the chances are you'll reach for an antihistamine. If eczema is irritating you, then some kind of skin cream, perhaps a steroid, will soothe you for a while. For asthma, inhalers are the most likely answer. All of these things can ease symptoms or reduce the risk of a reaction, but none can cure the condition. No tablet, cream or puffer will eradicate the cause. And, as most of us know to our cost, all these medications have side effects, some of them extremely unpleasant. Most important of all, none of them can get to the root of the problem. None can communicate with the immune system.

So, could probiotics be one of the keys to strengthening that system and reducing the risk of allergy and asthma?

What is an allergy?

Allergy is the word we use to define an abnormal response to a normal substance, an overreaction of the body's immune system either to something in the atmosphere or to a particular food or food ingredient. One extreme example is the violent reaction some people experience when exposed to just the tiniest amount of nuts.

This acute allergic response, or IgE, can lead to anaphylaxis, which is life threatening. At the other end of the scale, however, many people experience a less acute reaction, known as food sensitivity, perhaps to dairy products or wheat, which might give them bloating or constipation, joint pain or migraines. There are many triggers for allergies and intolerances, and it seems that we are becoming more and more sensitive to foods and other particles we are in contact with.

Have we reached allergy overload?

We know that an immune system supported by healthy intestines and beneficial bacteria should be able to deal quietly and efficiently with any 'invasion' so that the person concerned is completely unaware of any problem. In other words, they are not allergic. But as a result of continual exposure to high levels of toxicity, stress and disturbed gut bacteria, there's a far greater likelihood of allergy or sensitivity occurring, because an already weakened immune system has become programmed to malfunction and overreact. The eventual outcome of such persistent pressure is the possibility of multiple allergic reactions. They call it system overload or total load concept: the probability that the severity of any reaction to, say, food, inhalants, chemicals, airborne dust or pollen will increase in direct proportion to the number of allergens to which the person is exposed.

The hygiene hypothesis

To explain the meteoric rise in allergies and asthma, science has put forward something called the hygiene hypothesis. Sounds complicated but it isn't.

The 'hygiene' viewpoint came from the idea that the relatively clean living conditions most of us are familiar with today have possibly prevented us during infancy from being colonised by the bacteria that we all need in order to develop a healthy immune system. It was based on studies that found hay fever and eczema were more common in homes with one child but far less so in youngsters from larger families who, it was assumed, would be exposed to more viruses and bacteria via their brothers or sisters. And where hygiene was considered a priority, there were found to be correspondingly higher levels of asthma, hay fever and allergic dermatitis. However, this doesn't help to explain why, in a family of several children, only one may be severely allergic while the others are never affected.

In our modern world, at least in countries considered 'developed', we're deluged with product advertising for specialised soaps, sprays, wipes, lotions and liquids, all targeted at keeping ourselves and our families free of (scary word coming up here) germs! But some experts are convinced that those same products are taking out good bugs too, compromising immune systems and destroying the natural equilibrium that helps protect children from disease.

Does this mean we should all give up washing our hands?

Definitely not! First of all, these observations relate specifically to babies and toddlers, and the belief that exposure during the early part of life, and especially before the age of six months, to the usual bacteria associated with growing up can help strengthen the immune system against allergic reactions. But there needs to be balance. It doesn't mean that it's good for all of us to start licking the floor, coughing and sneezing all over others, picking our noses or snogging the dog.

Never forget that the kinds of bacteria we can acquire from these and other sources can also cause disease. Lack of basic hygiene, especially regular hand washing, is believed to be a major contributing factor to the rapid spread of superbugs (see page 123). More diligent use of soap and hot water will neither harm our immune systems (more likely it will help) nor increase the likelihood of succumbing to allergies.

Let's look at the research

The study that kicked off the hygiene hypothesis talked about exposure to what we would perhaps consider 'bad' bacteria but not at the role of friendly flora in boosting the immune system. When the idea was first proposed, in 1989, research concerning probiotics was very much in its infancy. But more recently, scientists are expanding the same theory to see how exposure to beneficial bacteria might affect human resistance to disease in general and to allergies in particular.

They're now looking beyond household cleanliness and considering other factors that could have a negative effect on the ability of a child's immune system to fight infection and, in particular, on the levels of friendly flora, both of which might explain the horrendously high levels of allergy-related conditions. These include the facility of babies being born by Caesarean section so that they don't have the benefit of picking up essential bacteria from the birth canal, coupled to the fact that, in many cases, breastfeeding is either done for a much shorter time than used to be the case or not done at all.

The other big issues

There are two other major events that upset the balance of good gut bugs and increase the risk of allergies.

One is the albatross of antibiotics

If you're expecting me to tell you that there's a connection between the risk of contracting allergies and the use of antibiotics, then you'd be right. It's rare indeed to find someone who says they have never needed to take antibiotics. Even one course can blow your good gut bugs to smithereens. The greater the number of courses, the greater the chance of conditions such as eczema, asthma and hay fever, but possibly food allergies too.

The other is a crap diet

Whoops! Sorry if you're offended in any way by my language, but I do need to get across to you, that eating rubbish does your gut flora no favours and could even be killing you. Why not take another look at the Good Gut Upgrade (Chapter 2) to see what improvements you might make?

In more detail . . .

Studies on the gut flora of tiny tots and toddlers have shown that those who already suffer with allergies tend to have lower levels of the beneficial *Bifidobacteria* and are more likely to carry harmful species such as *Clostridium difficile* and *Staphylococcus aureus*, especially in bottle-fed infants. Other studies, too, are consistent in finding lower levels of good gut bugs in those with allergies.

It seems likely that where there is a lack of beneficial bacteria in early life, the immune system doesn't mature properly and, as a result, it overreacts to the invaders, which causes allergies. On the other hand, helpful gut flora stimulate the immune system and 'train' it to get it ready so that it reacts efficiently when it's needed.

Several studies show that babies and toddlers whose diets were supplemented with the right kind of probiotic had significantly less risk of developing eczema, a condition often associated with allergy. Probiotics have also been used to control eczema and cow's milk allergy. In studies where probiotics were given to babies in their formula feed or to nursing mothers directly, there was an important reduction in intestinal inflammation, which tied in with a significant lessening of the symptoms of eczema.

Researchers suggest that probiotic bacteria may promote a protective barrier in patients with eczema and food allergy, and by alleviating intestinal inflammation, may act as a useful tool in the treatment of food allergy. In other words, exposure to good gut bugs early in life could make the chance of contracting allergy-related diseases much less likely. And there seems no doubt now that the likelihood of atopic eczema occurring in high-risk infants could be reduced by using probiotics. For many years, I've been recommending probiotics as part of the dietary support for allergy patients and find that, in most cases, it makes a very big difference indeed, significantly reducing the risk of reaction. The most remarkable improvements have been in children with asthma and eczema and for babies suffering with full-body eczema who had previously been swathed in cotton bandages and mittens.

Also encouraging are reports that adults who take regular yoghurt drinks, yoghurt or probiotic supplements have fewer symptoms of allergic rhinitis (runny nose caused by allergies).

Action plan for allergies

Arm yourself against getting an allergy by following the suggestions below:

1 Get tested. If you're concerned that you may have an allergy, find an experienced and qualified clinical ecologist, nutritionist or allergy specialist who has a proven track record in treating asthma, eczema and food allergies, and can carry out a range of recognised tests, including those for candidiasis and leaky gut syndrome. See Resources for labs who do testing.

2 Cut your allergen exposure. Protect yourself as much as you can from allergy aggravators such as house-dust mite. Air the bedclothes in between washes, as often as weather permits. Clean under the bed at least once a week. Use mattress and pillow protectors. Use microfibre cloths such as E-cloths, which clean and polish without chemicals. Avoid strong chemical-based household cleaning fluids. Don't use carpet deodorants, perfumes and stick-on, plug-in or spray air fresheners. Change to environmentally friendly, biodegradable washing products that are phosphate and perfume-free. For washing-machine use, try Eco-Ball or Turbo Plus. These hypoallergenic discs work without the use of detergent by ionising the water that then attracts dirt from the clothes. Reusable for several hundred washes, they won't lift really ingrained dirt but are excellent for everyday washing. A lot of sufferers are allergic to fabric softener but reusable tumble-dryer balls are a great alternative.

3 Check your salt loading. Salt can make allergics more reactive to histamine. It's easy to reach excess because so much salt is hidden in packaged and processed foods. The only way to cut back is to rely less on packets and cans. When you do go for convenience, at least make sure you read the labels and choose items that are low in salt or salt-free.

4 Invest in a daily, best-quality multivitamin–mineral to top up any nutrients missing from the diet and provide additional immune-system support. Some vitamins such as B_6 and C have natural antihistamine activity. In one study, vitamin B_{12} was shown to reduce asthma symptoms. An open-minded GP may be willing to prescribe a course of monthly injections. If not, go for a good-quality B_{12} supplement that is separate from your multi-vitamin. Other research confirms that ginkgo biloba can ease con-striction in asthma. Lignans (see page 96) and omegas-3 and 6 essential fatty acids may also be useful for eczema. I have successfully used both alongside probiotics.

5 Take Dr Vogel's Echinaforce. It's usually recommended for colds, but it can be a very useful supplement for dampening allergies too. Start taking it at least two months before your allergy season begins. More details on page 189.

6 Take probiotics during pregnancy. There's good evidence that doing so can help reduce the risk of eczema in the newborn. And carry on taking probiotics during breastfeeding. One study in particular has shown that taking probiotics during pregnancy and breastfeeding may lessen the risk of a mum who is already an allergy sufferer passing on her allergic tendencies to her breastfed baby.

If you're pregnant or planning a family, make every effort to breastfeed. It's long been known that babies who are breastfed seem to be better protected from asthma in childhood and adult-hood than those who receive only formula. If breastfeeding isn't an option for you, then talk to the paediatrician about the use of probiotics in formula. If you or your partner, or anyone in your immediate family, has a known intolerance to cow's milk, then it could be worth considering using Nanny Goat Formula (see Resources) for your baby and adding probiotics to that. (See also Chapter 22.)

7 Enjoy a daily probiotic drink. People who include fermented milk products in their diet are likely to have a better immunity to pollen. Research tells us that sufferers of seasonal allergies who took a regular probiotic drink containing *Lactobacillus casei* over a five-month period had lower levels of a particular antibody that tends to aggravate allergy symptoms. They also had higher levels of a different antibody, called IgG, which is believed to protect against allergic reactions.

8 Add probiotic supplements to your regular diet. The research so far makes a very good case for taking probiotics – supported by a good diet – to help ease the symptoms of respiratory allergies and also for asthma and eczema.

Strengthening the gut with probiotics

There is no doubt that certain probiotics have the ability to control the inflammation associated with allergic reactions and, where probiotics have been given to babies and toddlers with eczema, there is good evidence of reduced adverse reactions to cow's milk. Friendly flora play an important part in strengthening the gut lining, which reduces the risk of leaky gut syndrome and therefore helps prevent unwanted food molecules getting into the bloodstream in the first place.

Be a patient patient

You may have been unwell for a long time. Good nutrition is powerful stuff, but don't expect it to work overnight. Supplemented nutrients can take anything from 12 to 16 weeks to make any improvements.

Very important point
Remember that we are all individual and that not everyone will respond to probiotic therapy. However, because these substances are considered safe to use under nearly all circumstances, I think it's mad not to try. Regular and consistent treatment is essential if you are going to get results. It's no good just following a course for a couple of weeks and then expecting miracles.

12.

Body Odour or Bad Breath?

At one time or another most of us have been on the receiving end of someone else's less than pleasant pongs. It might be cheesy feet, acrid underarms, honky halitosis or the room-emptying consequences of a bit of furtive farting. Some people might be offended by such a situation, others might feel sorry for the person concerned, but would it ever occur to anyone that the perpetrator might have a health problem? Probably not, but that's exactly what it could be. Body odour is very often a sign that all is not well.

What's to blame?

Although it's true that smelly skin could simply be the result of a reluctance to make contact with soap and water, and bad breath might easily be cured by investing in a new toothbrush and some regular flossing, it's nevertheless the case that most body odours are down to bad bacteria. The reason that armpits, groins and other sweaty sites get whiffy is because bacteria like to grow in warm, dark, damp locations. It can happen to anyone. If you've ever noticed strong, unpleasant odours emanating not only from your waste products but perhaps also from your feet, groin or underarms, you can bet that, one way or another, it'll be the result of bad bacteria having a fine old time, multiplying, decomposing and blowing a few raspberries to celebrate. It's worth pointing out here that if your internal ecology is up the creek, then the bacteria on your skin is, almost certainly, going to be out of balance, too.

My own experience in clinic suggests that patients with these kinds of problems generally have poor digestion and an overgrowth of undesirable bacteria in the gut. Improving the digestion and introducing regular doses of probiotics alongside a healthy prebiotic diet almost always corrects the problem. In very severe cases where someone is suffering from socially inhibiting body odour, a probiotic programme can be enhanced by a course of cleansing herbs and/or colonic irrigation.

Flatulent emissions

One of the most common 'scent' problems that people suffer, and the one that they're probably least likely to tell their doctor about, is gas – otherwise known as burping, belching, blowing off or farting. All this comes under the general heading of flatus, which is defined as 'gas generated in the stomach or intestines' or, more kindly, 'a puff or blast of wind'. Flatulence by the way is the noun used to describe the tendency to windiness, usually taken to indicate the distension of the stomach or bowels by gases formed during digestion.

How often you belch, rumble or fart – and how sweet you smell (or don't) – may also depend to a very large extent on your probiotic status; in other words, whether or not you have enough good bugs to keep the stinky brigade under control.

If body odour is a problem for you or your nearest and dearest, the dietary and other advice contained in the Good Gut Upgrade (Chapter 2) and Chapter 4 may be of particular help.

Bad breath

Halitosis or bad breath (doctors call it oral malodour) is believed to affect up to half of the human adult population. Although we don't usually think about it as being a medical condition, it is, nevertheless, a sign of imbalance either in the mouth (teeth, gums or tongue) or in the stomach.

Malodour can be caused by rotting teeth, unhealthy gums, a dicky digestion, the ulcer bacteria *Helicobacter pylori* or any number of other illnesses. For the moment, let's just look at the oral cavity and especially the gums and the tongue, the main source of smelly bacteria in an otherwise healthy mouth.

It's a fact, it's gum disease, not tooth decay, that's the biggest cause of tooth loss. In the UK alone, gum disease is said to affect 75 per cent of the population over the age of 35. Half of all teenagers have some form of gum disease and only 60 per cent of women aged 45 can claim to have all their own teeth! Scarier still is the fact that smoking causes 50 per cent of all cases of gum disease. Poor dental hygiene is also linked to high alcohol intake and, most obviously, to lots of sweet and sugary foods in the diet, all of which can make life difficult for otherwise supportive oral bacteria.

It's a comfy location if you happen to be a vandalistic bacterium on the lookout to make mischief. If you are a smelly old mouth bug you can feed on the almost constant supply of food that your host pushes into his or her mouth every day. And your particular human, the one you live with, seems to be addicted to the same types of grub that you also really enjoy – so why move on? When you've had a really good feed on all that starchy stuff that's stuck around the place and you've spat out a sack-load of cavity-causing acid, you can hide away while you wait for the next meal. No one will notice you, even if you sit on your owner's front tooth, because you can glue yourself invisibly to the static that's been created by a mucusy film, called plaque, which builds up so conveniently every time a meal shows up. And while you're lurking under the adhesive remains of your human provider's lunchtime sandwich, you can chat to all your other malcontent mates who are busily weaving a web of bacterial chains all around the mouth.

Of course all you bad bacteria know that plaque, if ignored and not cleaned out every day, can lead to diseased gums and holes in your host's teeth. But, hey, why would you care? You were born to cause cavities.

Did you know?

Cavities (which dentists call 'caries') are caused when the acid that's produced by bacteria feeding on starches and sugars in the mouth attack the enamel, slowly eating away at the mineral surface until it breaks through the inner layer, the dentine, and then the deeper parts of the tooth known as the pulp. Once inside, the bacteria set up home among the blood vessels and nerves, leading to you needing a root canal filling or an extraction.

Mouth bugs are opportunists and will take any chance they can get to crawl deeper into our tissues, such as during dental surgery, and could cause other serious health problems including damage to the heart. In someone with an already weakened immunity or in diabetes, for example, even normally harmless bacteria can become troublesome.

Fillings or no fillings?

Ever wondered why it is that some people never seem to need dental treatment and others have mouths full of fillings? There are a number of reasons:

1 Saliva. Some body types produce loads of saliva, which certainly contributes towards plaque control. Firstly because it helps to wash some of the plaque away and also because saliva contains small amounts of a natural antibiotic and a starch-digesting enzyme called amylase. People who suffer with desert-dry mouths have to work harder at their oral hygiene because bad bacteria build up more easily where saliva is in short supply. This may be just an unfortunate natural occurrence, but it is made worse by smoking, heavy drinking, certain drugs and medical treatments. Unfortunately, dry-mouth sufferers often try to work up saliva by sucking sweets or sipping sodas, not realising that they're simply adding welcome sugar supplies to an existing bacterial bonanza!

2 Sugar. Mouth bugs love anything that's even remotely related to sugar, so how much carbohydrate (sugary and starchy foods, such as bread, biscuits, cake, and so on) you have in your diet can determine how likely you are to succumb to collections of cavities or honky halitosis.

3 Clean teeth. Obviously, dental hygiene makes a massive difference. If you allow acid-producing pathogens to inhabit your mouth and you don't do anything about keeping them under control, then the result is going to be a mouth full of fillings or false teeth. Or if your dentist remains on your list of Persons to Ignore, then you might already have a mouth of rotting teeth and camel's breath.

4 Protective bacteria. A few lucky souls are simply blessed with very low numbers of pathogenic bacteria and far higher levels of protective bacteria. The results of extensive research in New Zealand suggests that those lucky people who never seem to suffer sore throats or bad breath – or for that matter rarely get sick with colds, flu or throat infections – may acquire a different set of mouth bugs, in particular a beneficial one called *Streptococcus salivarius* K12, which is closely related to *Streptococcus thermophilus* used in the manufacture of some yoghurts. *S. salivarius* K12 works because, incredibly, it can 'sense' invading bacteria, whereupon it fires naturally produced antibiotic agents at the bad bugs, puncturing them and causing them to leak and die. Isn't nature incredible?

Sadly, only 2 per cent of the population fall into this auspicious category, so it follows that 98 per cent are missing this must-have microorganism. Why? Well, in the first place, it's probably down to heredity. Where the right conditions prevail, the first sign of *S. salivarius* will be in babies who acquire it from their mothers soon after birth. But if Mum doesn't have any, then that won't happen. In addition, this helpful bacteria can't survive where there are low levels of oxygen or in an acid environment (a healthy mouth is slightly alkaline, otherwise all your teeth would fall out) so it isn't effective in cases of poor mouth hygiene. It would also struggle to survive in the mouth of a heavy drinker, smoker or sugar addict. Like all friendly microflora, it needs support, not neglect.

Did you know?
In the elderly, poor oral health can mean poor resistance to infection and involuntary weight loss simply because gum disease or dental difficulties are preventing them from eating and/or chewing properly. If you have an elderly relative or know a senior citizen who has these problems, encourage them to talk to their doctor or health visitor.

Action plan to beat bad mouth bugs

Keep the bad bacteria at bay by following the suggestions below:

1 Control the plaque. It can stick around like superglue, impervious to even the most aggressive tongue licking. The only real answer is to get busy with the toothbrush and the floss after meals and spit it out. The mechanical clean-out will remove far more bugs than any antibacterial mouthwash.

2 Brush your tongue or use a tongue scraper. This is where most people's bad-breath problems originate. Certain bacteria here break down proteins in foods and from your body, and have stinky by-products.

3 Avoid regular chemical mouthwash products which contain alcohol, because they can dry out your mouth. If you find that you have a dry mouth anyway, which makes you drink a lot more water, then there may be an underlying problem with mouth bacteria or rhinitis (see below).

Top Tip

Unfortunately, it can be difficult to tell if your own breath is bad and most of us are reluctant to ask someone else! If you smoke, drink a lot of coffee, eat a lot of red meat, suffer with regular bouts of acidity, haven't flossed or cleaned your teeth since this morning or if your mouth feels like the bottom of a birdcage, the chances are pretty high that you'll not be nice to be near. A useful way to check is to lick your forearm and then sniff the result. If it honks, then floss if possible – or at least go get some mouthwash! Remember that bad digestion and bacterial overgrowth in the gut can also cause bad breath.

---

4 If you constantly have to clear the throat, it may be being caused by postnasal drip, where proteins from your sinuses are dripping down onto your tongue and are 'feeding' the problem bacteria. Problems like this one and the 'dry mouth syndrome' may require a trip to a professional.

5 Find a good-quality natural toothpaste. If you prefer products that are free from Triclosan and sodium lauryl sulphate (SLS), which can cause allergies and skin problems for some people, try Comvita's Toothgel or Fennel Toothpaste from the Green People Company.

6 Use a mouthwash every day. Again, if possible, choose one that's SLS-free. Green People Fennel Mouthwash or Neem Mouthwash from Xynergy Health Products are both effective and good for regular use. Kiwiherb mouthwash is high strength (not one for anybody who grimaces at strong tastes) and needs to be diluted but probably has few equals in terms of its antimicrobial effects. Bear in mind, though, that mouthwash products, however good they are, will only have a temporary effect.

7 Clean your teeth after breakfast and your evening meal. If you can't do the toothpaste thing after lunch, at least use mouthwash or swill the mouth with water to dislodge as much gunge as possible. The same applies if you have eaten fresh fruit or juice – it's still a tooth-damaging carbohydrate even though it's good for you.

8 Consider a course of Xylotene, which is derived from d-xylose. Xylose belongs to a food group known as glyconutrients or nutritional sugars. This type of sugar is 'tooth-friendly' because it doesn't cause decay, can reduce sensitivity and help remineralisation of teeth. If you have gum disease, sensitivity, dry mouth or other tooth problems, add a small amount (no more than a level teaspoon) to a glass of water and rinse your mouth with it. Swallow it; don't spit it out. D-xylose is often hailed as a beneficial one-off treatment for mouth ulcers because, if you put a spoonful of the powder directly onto the ulcer and hold it there until it dissolves, the ulcer itself often disappears completely in less than a day. It can also be used as a sugar substitute, being as sweet as ordinary table sugar but with 40 per cent of the calories (see Resources).

> **! Very important point**
> If you use xylose-based products, take care not to exceed the recommend dose. It's generally recognised as safe and has many claimed benefits but, as with several other sugar substitutes, in particular sorbitol, it can have a decidedly laxative effect if you take too much! There's more information on glyconutrients in the section on urinary health – page 236.

9 Watch your intake of sugary snacks, for example, biscuits, chocolate, sweets, cake, those oddly named 'soft' drinks (they're still hard on your teeth) and sugar in your beverages.

10 Chew all your food really thoroughly. This helps to reduce the amount that gets stuck around the gums and also encourages saliva production.

11 Get yourself checked for *Helicobacter pylori*.

12 If you've been affected by gum disease, especially where there is a problem with loose teeth or gingivitis, then consider the use of a good-quality supplement of coenzyme Q_{10} (CoQ_{10}), also sometimes called quinone (not quinine). Studies show that CoQ_{10}, which is probably best known as a heart supplement, can be extremely effective in fighting gum disease, strengthening gums, stopping bleeding and clearing up infection. Small doses of CoQ_{10} (less than 30mg), such as those found in some multi supplements, may not be strong enough to make a significant difference. And be aware that there are quite a lot of not-so-good brands on the market. I usually recommend Pharma Nord Bio-Quinone 30mg at two or three capsules a day until the situation has resolved. This product, which has a significant amount of research behind it, is also an excellent heart-health supplement.

13 If you're a smoker, a coffee drinker or you eat a lot of curries and other spicy food, be aware that other people might not enjoy the after-effects. Improving your nice-to-be-near status is really easy: wash your mouth out after eating, carry portable mini-toothbrushes in your purse or pocket and invest in some breath fresheners.

14 Boost your good gut bugs by adding fermented milk products, such as buttermilk, kefir or live yoghurt to your diet every day.

15 Take a regular probiotic supplement (see page 265). There's good evidence that it helps to regulate the growth of troublesome bacteria, reducing the risk of dental decay in children's teeth, making for fewer adult cavities and lessening the likelihood of mouth ulcers and other oral infections. Probiotics, together with a healthy diet, can help us in our fight against tooth decay and gum disease, and could also reduce our risk of throat and respiratory infections.

16 Treat yourself to mouth-care products that contain *Streptococcus salivarius* K12. It's being marketed in throat lozenges and as part of a dental package aimed at maintaining oral health and treating halitosis. It's available around the world under a variety of different brand names. Visit www.blis.co.nz for regularly updated information.

Action plan to beat BO

Smell sweet by following the suggestions below:

1 Improve your digestion. When the body doesn't break food down or deal with it efficiently, one of the results can be bad smells. Make a start right now by sitting down to meals, taking your time, never eating on the move and chewing every mouthful thoroughly.

2 Upgrade your diet. Including more of the right kinds of fibre (page 103) and choosing a selection of the prebiotic foods on page 85 will help give healthy support to the intestines, which sustain the production of your 'in-house' friendly bacteria.

3 Cut back on red meat, especially beef and pork. People who eat a lot of meat often have the least desirable body perfume!

4 Forget wheat bran-based breakfast cereals and change to oats.

5 Avoid sugar.

6 Drink plenty of water between meals. But keep in mind what I said about dry mouth syndrome and see your dentist and doctor if it's a problem.

7 Wear natural fabrics. Avoid non-breathable fibres next to the skin.

8 Avoid ordinary soap. Many basic types of soap, especially cheaper brands, can be quite alkaline, disturbing the skin's natural pH (acid balance), thereby encouraging odorous bacteria to multiply. Check the label and choose products that are pH balanced.

9 Don't be faithful to just one brand of deodorant. The body can become sensitive to it, or get used to it. Ring the changes and try to go for those that are least likely to disturb the body's natural pH and bacterial balance. Try natural 'crystal' deodorants or any others that are free from harsh chemicals and perfumes. You'll find different brands in your pharmacy or health shop (also see Resources).

10 Take a regular probiotic supplement. It really can make a big difference between smelling sweet and smelling stale.

13.

Cholesterol and Other Heart-disease Risk Factors

Although you may think that the link between high cholesterol and heart disease is written in scientific stone never to be questioned, you might be surprised to learn that it's still surrounded by much controversy. There's certainly good evidence that neither saturated fat nor the cholesterol in food has any detrimental effect on cholesterol levels in the blood. Indeed, some leading experts are on record as saying that fretting about cholesterol levels is barking up entirely the wrong tree and that by paying it so much attention, we're ignoring other, perhaps more important, risk factors. Before we talk about some of the less well known things that are thought to affect our heart health, let's look at the current favourite of the drug companies – cholesterol.

If my clinical experience is anything to go by, high cholesterol is teetering on the brink of becoming an epidemic. The great sadness is that, for many, it's a self-inflicted wound. Yes, of course there are a small number of people who suffer with the type of cholesterol problem that runs in families, called familial hypercholesterolaemia, but for the majority diet may be entirely to blame.

Going down a blind alley to beat cholesterol

For the majority who are referred to my clinic with elevated cholesterol, the patient pattern is nearly always the same. Although I see plenty of people who are eating an appalling diet, low in vegetables and fruit, and overloaded with fry-ups and takeaways, a lot of patients are already trying very hard indeed to avoid what they believe to be unhealthy foods. They drink skimmed milk, eat zero-fat yoghurts, always choose low-fat polyunsaturates or buy spreads that come with a cholesterol-lowering pledge. They avoid things like Brazil nuts, walnuts, sunflower seeds or avocado pear, because they think these will either make them put on weight or increase their fat loading, pushing their cholesterol up (it won't). For the same reason, they steer clear of eggs as if they were a plague (it's a myth, by the way, since there's no evidence that eggs cause a problem). They'll buy sunflower oil because they think it's lower in fat or better for their cholesterol than olive oil (it isn't). They would never think of using coconut milk because it's branded as an evil saturate (even though it's good for you). And because they've read an article or heard someone say that dietary fibre helps reduce cholesterol levels, they plough dutifully through bowls of sugar-laden bran each breakfast time (yes, it is sugar-laden, even if you don't add sugar). And yet, their cholesterol levels – and very often also their triglycerides (blood fats) – stay stubbornly above normal.

By the time they get to see me, they're either already taking statins or some other cholesterol-lowering drug, or are on the verge of doing so. They're also often on the edge of desperation.

Surprising advice

The dietary guidance that I give them sometimes provokes surprise and a good deal of relief and pleasure when they discover that the unsustaining and tasteless diet they've been trying so hard to stick to for months or years (and which hasn't actually been working) may no longer be necessary. I realise that to many people what I'm about to tell you will sound like heresy but I've been doing this job for more than 20 years and have such persistently good results with patients who present with high cholesterol and high blood fats (often very high indeed) that I can't ignore the feedback.

Before we look at some of the best things we can do to help our heart and circulation, let's first of all consider:

What exactly is cholesterol?

When we talk about cholesterol, most of us tend to think of it blocking up our arteries and thereby risking our imminent demise. It's probably for this reason that it's so often seen as the arch villain of the heart-disease saga when, in fact, cholesterol is a vital health-promoting substance that none of us could manage without. Cholesterol plays a key role in the manufacture of hormones and cell membranes. It's needed for the growth and development of our brains and nervous system and for vitamin D production. And it gets involved when there's any healing to be done in the body. It has even been suggested that the reason cholesterol shows up where there is scarring of the arteries is because it's there in its repairing capacity.

Is there more to clogged arteries than just cholesterol?

Definitely! OK, so the received wisdom is that high cholesterol levels are caused by eating too much saturated fat. The most oft-quoted research to support this view is something known as The Framingham Heart Study, which was begun in 1948 and involved more than 5,000 people living in and around the town of Framingham in Massachusetts. Regarded now as a gold-standard piece of research, the work extended over four decades, involved three generations of participants and investigated many different aspects of cardiovascular research, including heart failure, high blood pressure, stroke, atherosclerosis and family history. The cholesterol issue was only one aspect of this long ongoing study but it's an area that has not been beyond criticism. In particular, there's the much-repeated and curious anomaly that the higher the intake of saturated fat, the lower the cholesterol reading!

It's my personal belief that there's far more to heart disease than simply how much cholesterol or fat there is in the bloodstream and that the present scourge of cardiovascular problems could have more to do with a number of other factors. One is inflammation (see page 254). Another, which used to be a top risk factor for heart disease but which has fallen out of favour since cholesterol took over the number-one slot, is stress. Consider how much excessive and negative stress we are all under these days and I think it's something we should reconsider. Also significant is the *change* in the type and quality of fats and oils that we now consume. We've swapped things like saturated butterfat, lard, dripping, tallow and chicken fat for polyunsaturated vegetable oil, much of it chemically processed and hydrogenated – but has it done any good? Apparently not.

Save us from the 'H' word

Hydrogenation is a process that is known to damage the beneficial *cis* fatty acids in the natural oils and turn some of them into trans-fatty acids (TFAs) which, once they get into our arteries, are considered to be a greater risk to cardiovascular disease than any other major food source, including saturates. Throughout the 1990s, I was writing regular articles on the likely damaging effects of hydrogenated oils for the national press and several magazines, and was repeatedly assured by margarine manufacturers that their products were entirely safe. Although they didn't appear to agree with me at the time that TFAs might be a potential health problem, it's interesting to note that product packaging these days often makes the claim 'low in trans-fatty acids'.

Trans-fats are not essential fats and they do not encourage good health. Official advice is that TFAs are harmful, even at low levels of consumption and should be avoided wherever possible. Thankfully, many products, especially supermarket own labels, no longer contain trans-fats. But it's worth being aware that any foods you eat that are fried in polyunsaturated oils, especially if the oil is used and re-used (watch out for takeaways), will have created their own trans-fats. And they aren't restricted to margarines and cooking oils. They turn up in a whole range of packaged foods, too, so it really is wise to read the labels and watch out for the H word. If the oil used is hydrogenated, then TFAs could be lurking.

How trans-fats affect your cholesterol levels

Trans-fats it seems, are thoroughly bad news. TFAs encourage fats and cholesterol to oxidise (corrode, like rusty tin) so that it becomes clingy and hard to shift. Then it gets collected up by white blood cells known as macrophages, which form deposits together with other fatty substances, calcium and bits of accumulated tissue, any of which can 'catch' or get caught up along the lining of the blood vessels. Sometimes they cement themselves right into the artery walls. This is what we call arterial plaque (doctors say atheroma, hence the medical term for this condition: atherosclerosis). Old plaque, not unlike an elderly knee joint, stiffens up with calcium deposits and is harder to move. Apart from the actual material, it's also common to find swelling or inflammation at these sites in the blood system, which can further contribute to any gridlock. In fact, some experts believe that inflammation could be a major cause of narrowing of the arteries. But it doesn't necessarily mean this will happen to you. Everybody has some kind of build-up, which can start to accumulate as early as one year of age and yet doesn't necessarily lead to heart attack or stroke in later life.

Could bacteria be a factor?

To suggest that bad bacteria could play a role in blocking arteries and causing heart disease may seem strange, especially as saturated fat and high cholesterol levels have so long been pilloried as the direct cause. But it's no more heretical than another idea that we all now accept as completely normal: that most digestive ulcers are the result of ...? Yes, bacteria.

As long ago as 1973 it was noticed that beneficial bacteria might be able to influence cholesterol levels. Since then, there's been a whole raft of research looking into whether or not adding friendly flora to the diet would help regulate both LDL (low-density lipoprotein – the bad cholesterol) and/or triglycerides (blood fats). Interestingly, as is always the way with scientific observation, a few showed no benefit, but other results have been very positive.

Most of the research work looking at the effects of probiotics on cholesterol has involved hens, mice, pigs, rabbits and rats, and – not surprisingly – has so far produced mixed results. But in humans, overall, it seems that beneficial bacteria can make modest yet worthwhile reductions in cholesterol levels. If you agree with the statistic that every 1 per cent drop in cholesterol equates to a 2–3 per cent reduction in the risk of contracting coronary heart disease, then the regular use of probiotics (in particular those containing *Lactobacillus acidophilus*), could, it seems, cut your own personal risk by anything up to 10 per cent.

One study used a dairy-free formula of fermented oatmeal combined with a fruit drink and a particular strain of friendly flora known as *Lactobacillus plantarum*. *L. plantarum* occurs naturally in the intestines and has been shown in animal studies to have several benefits, including supporting the lining of the gut, reducing gut wall inflammation, improving liver function and benefiting the immune system. In humans, this same strain was found to lessen the abdominal bloating so common in people suffering irritable bowel syndrome. But of particular interest here is the fact that it also decreased concentrations of a substance called fibrinogen. This may sound completely unrelated to the subject in hand but actually it's quite important. Fibrinogen is a protein in the blood that reacts with other substances to form blood clots. Although not always tested unless there are serious indications of cardiovascular disease, my experience has been that fibrinogen may be a problem even when cholesterol is normal.

Be aware!

What's now certain is that there's much more to heart-attack risk than just having elevated cholesterol and that, if you're aware of those risks, you're much better placed to do something about them. Although there are plenty of drugs available to lower cholesterol, there are also a multitude of other factors to consider. Apart from your triglycerides and the fibrinogen, your risk rating goes up considerably if you suffer with any of the following (many of which can be improved by a better diet):

High blood pressure (hypertension).

High levels of glucose in the blood, affecting not only diabetics but also those in a pre-diabetic state.

Elevated homocysteine. If this toxic by-product is allowed to accumulate in your circulatory system, it can scuff and scar the walls of your arteries and make it easier for plaque to get caught up, just as waste might in a drainpipe that wasn't perfectly smooth along all of its surface. Although most blood test results will tell you that between 5 and 15 millimoles per litre of blood (5–15 mmol/l) are OK, research suggests that the chances of a heart attack rise steeply if homocysteine rises above 6 mmol/l. One cardiologist told me that he thought the healthiest level of homocysteine should be nearer zero! (And by the way, high homocysteine is also considered to be a serious risk factor for Alzheimer's disease.) In most cases, excesses can be sorted by taking a good-quality multivitamin supplement that contains all the B-complex nutrients, especially folic acid and vitamins B_6 and B_{12}. Studies show that this can also be helpful even in advanced stages of atherosclerosis.

Lipoprotein-a is a substance made up of sticky fatty particles, which encourages clots to form in the blood. It is rarely tested. Likewise, another substance known as VLDL (very low-density lipoprotein) also contributes to blood clotting.

C-reactive protein is a protein that is produced in response to inflammation. Interestingly, it's been found to rise in people whose diets contain trans-fats. Elevated C-reactive protein is now considered to be a good indicator of heart-attack risk *even if cholesterol levels are normal*. It's suggested that someone with a C-RP reading above 3mg per litre of blood (3mg/l) could be three times more likely to suffer a heart attack. People with low C-RP scores, however, have the lowest risk.

Red cell magnesium. This is one of the most important minerals in the fight against hypertension, heart disease and stroke and, if it's low, you could be more susceptible to heart and circulatory problems.

Serum vitamin E is the reading that tells you how much vitamin

E is in your blood. Having too little can increase your risk of heart disease.

Ongoing mental and emotional stress can increase your risk of cardiovascular disease, even if all your blood test results are normal.

Bad bacteria. Researchers have found that atherosclerotic lesions (the damaged bits in the arteries) contain pathogenic bacteria; among them, *Chlamydophila* (sometimes written *Chlamydia*) *pneumoniae*, a major trigger for pneumonia, bronchitis and pharyngitis, and *Porphyromonas gingivalis*, the primary cause of gum disease. Apparently, they get into the blood by 'hitch-hiking' on lipid (fat) cells. In addition, where there are repeated or chronic infections such as bronchitis or tooth abscesses, or in smokers, small amounts of bacteria sometimes find their way into the bloodstream and settle in the artery walls. Although giving antibiotics to people with these bacteria has not shown any reduction in heart attack, experts do believe that this discovery adds further weight to the neglected theory that some cases of heart disease could be caused by infection.

Meanwhile, don't forget what we've learned throughout *Good Gut Bugs* about pathogenic bacteria: the risk of them causing us damage is likely to be far less if we regularly replenish our supportive friendly flora.

What about blood pressure?

I think there are enough good results from studies showing that probiotics may be valuable as part of the treatment of high blood pressure to warrant including them in the diet both as supplements and foods. It's been suggested that the fermentation process may be particularly important. It wouldn't be at all fair to give the impression that probiotics or fermented foods are a cure-all for people with hypertension but, once again, my experience with patients leads me to the view that they should be a fundamentally important part of treatment.

Action plan for cholesterol and other heart-disease factors

Help yourself fight cholesterol and other heart-disease problems by following the suggestions below:

1 Follow as much of the Good Gut Upgrade (Chapter 2) as you possibly can. This dietary information has proved in practice to be extremely helpful in lowering both cholesterol and blood pressure. In particular:

- Check your fat intake. It's not fat per se that's the villain but the type of fat you choose that's important. Watch out for processed fats, such as tubs of polyunsaturates, and foods that contain hydrogenated oils, and remember what I said about checking labels. While it may be wise to keep milk to a minimum and butter to sensible levels, there is good evidence that quality aged cheeses can be helpful in providing valuable probiotics to the diet.

- Don't let food manufacturers and supermarkets dictate your fat intake. Low-fat or diet versions of any particular food are nearly always more expensive than the plain unadulterated equivalent, and it's very possible that you'll go for low-fat polyunsaturates, zero-fat yoghurts, low-fat mayo or reduced-fat cheese, because you believe them to be helpful. But bear in mind that many of these will be processed in some way and could contain heavy doses of flavouring, preservatives, emulsifiers or stabilisers, some or all of which were added to replace the fat that was taken out. Some low-fat foods are simply that and remain additive-free, which is fine. But if the full-fat version is the only one that seems to be unadulterated, have you ever considered that it may actually be better to go for that and eat less of it? I remain convinced that a tub of full-fat live yoghurt, free of chemical concoctions is far healthier than the low-fat processed alternative.

- Don't be conned into thinking that cholesterol-lowering spreads are the answer to all your problems. I've met people who believe that because they're using one of these products, they can get away with an otherwise high-fat diet. The main reason for the success of such spreads is the inclusion of plant sterols, which have been shown in some studies to help lower cholesterol. Not all countries have endorsed their use as a food additive, however, and there have been a number of dissenting voices warning of potential dangers, in particular that sterols disturb the hormonal system and affect the absorption of beta-carotene and vitamin E. Something else rarely publicised is the official advice that patients who are already on statins should not use products containing plant sterols without first discussing this with their doctor.

Margarine was never a healthy food, even though the advertising might suggest otherwise, nor has it ever been recommended by government health departments as an essential component of a healthy diet. While processed plant sterols may be useful in small amounts, the products they're put into can still contain hydrogenated oils and a lorry-load of additives. Nearly every patient that I see in clinic is buying into the idea because they think they're helping themselves to a healthier cholesterol level. If you like 'sterol spreads' and can afford them, especially if you think that they're making a difference, then take no notice of me. But if I was your nutritionist, I would suggest that you saved your money and used other 'spready' things like small amounts of ripe avocado, hummus and even unsalted butter instead. By the way, natural plant sterols are found in abundance in a lot of the foods that you gave up because you thought they were going to raise your cholesterol, especially in nuts and seeds, which also provide other important nutrients and dietary fibre!

- Cut out as much sugar (and sugary foods) as you can bear; diets high in the wrong kind of fat are definitely not good, but those that contain bad fats and sugars together are far worse.

- Don't get paranoid about foods that contain cholesterol, such as eggs. Research confirms what a lot of us have long suspected: eggs in the diet do not raise blood cholesterol by any significant degree and do not contribute to heart disease. Unless you are actually allergic to eggs or simply don't like them, free-range eggs provide valuable nutrients that will do you no harm.

- Include plenty of fibrous and prebiotic foods in your diet. This can improve both your blood fat and blood pressure levels. The lists on pages 85 and 103 will give you plenty of good ideas.

- Introduce a helping of daily flaxseed and make it a regular part of your new diet. Choose your flaxseed carefully. Low-priced products rarely contain the active ingredients that you need. (Full details are on page 97.)

- It's well worth including a probiotic yoghurt or probiotic drink of some kind every day, but check packaging details and make sure that they contain live cultures. Kefir (see page 86) is particularly good; if you don't like the taste, look upon it as an essential medicine and disguise the flavour with honey or fruit juice.

- Drink more water. It increases the blood volume which can help balance blood pressure.

- Cut back on alcohol. Although the recommendation that a glass of red wine is good for you remains true, excess alcohol can be a killer.

- Do whatever you can to avoid cigarette smoke – yours and other people's. Heart disease has long been linked to smoking, but now the infection theory has been resurrected, researchers are looking again at the possibility that, if you live with a smoker, you're more likely to pick up the very bacteria that are known as the 'primary candidates for causing atherosclerosis'. If you can't avoid exposure, then at least do everything possible to boost your immunity. Most important of all, look after your good gut bugs, because these are the best defence you have against unwanted bacteria.

- Protect yourself against that 'internal rusting' I was talking about earlier. This includes eating the healthiest possible diet, rich in antioxidant-loaded fresh fruit and vegetables, and taking a daily multivitamin–mineral supplement that – at the very least – contains carotenoids, B_2, B_6, B_{12}, folic acid, magnesium, selenium, zinc and vitamins C and E.

!

Very important points

- Always take your multi supplements with food, halfway through a meal, not at the beginning or the end, and never on an empty stomach.
- If you are prescribed warfarin/heparin or some other blood-thinning agent, check with your GP before taking supplements.

2 Go for regular checkups. When you have your cholesterol tested, remember that cholesterol readings tell you very little and may cause you to panic unnecessarily. Try to get readings for triglycerides, fibrinogen, homocysteine and C-reactive protein. And ask for your blood pressure to be checked at the same time. If your cholesterol is only slightly elevated but everything else is within normal limits, there may be no need at all for you to take a cholesterol-lowering drug.

3 If your blood pressure reading is high, make sure that it's taken at least three times, standing, sitting and lying down, and repeated over a three-day period before any decisions are made as to medication. It's very easy to assume from a single test that you have elevated blood pressure when there are many reasons for isolated high readings; for example, it may simply be that you were rushing before the appointment or were under particular stress that day.

4 If you have to take cholesterol-lowering drugs, don't allow them to give you a false sense of security. I remember a guest at a Sunday lunch party looking across the table at me over the top of his very rich dessert and saying, 'I don't suppose you approve of this, but it's all right, I'm on statins.' I've met lots of people who think that the protection offered by statins means they are then in some way immune from heart attack, stroke, thrombosis and other related conditions and, as a result, can throw dietary caution to the wind. Even if statins suit you (and they're not for everyone because, sometimes, the side effects are tough to take), they will only work for the time that you're using them, and while they may offer some protection they're certainly not a cure. Some people take them and still have high cholesterol.

5 If you're already on these drugs, bear in mind that they cause deficiencies of an important nutrient known as coenzyme Q_{10}, which is needed by the body for a healthy heart. Many experts now recommend that patients taking statins should also take a daily supplement of CoQ_{10}. There are many products on the market, but the one I have found most effective, and which has considerable research behind it, is Bio-Quinone 30mg produced by Pharma Nord of Denmark (see Resources). Recent unpublished work also suggests that statins can have a negative impact on gut flora.

Although I don't go along with the idea that statins should be given to everyone on a just-in-case basis, for some people medication may be the only option. But for real and lasting results you will nearly always need to make fundamental changes to your lifestyle and eating habits. In fact, nutritional support can be so effective that it's really worth trying to lower your cholesterol through diet *first* and to look upon medication as a *last* resort.

6 Do whatever you can to improve the way you deal with stress. It's still way up there in the league of heart-disease risk factors and has many more damaging effects on the body than there is space to mention here. I think it's worth noting, though, that stress hormones not only thicken the blood but they can also have a detrimental effect on gut flora.

7 Consider introducing a course of really good-quality probiotic supplements along with those important dietary changes. They have been shown to have many benefits. But please remember that probiotics alone are unlikely to provide the improvement that you can get by using them in conjunction with the healthy-eating recommendations contained in this chapter and in Chapter 2.

14.

Colds, Flu and Respiratory Infections

Did you know that studies carried out with healthy people show that those who use probiotic supplements and probiotic foods have fewer colds and winter infections, and as a result need to take fewer days off work? There's also good evidence to show that probiotics can be of real value in boosting and supporting a flagging immune system and in helping us to stay healthy. We also know that friendly flora have the power to:

- Prime (prepare) the immune system and increase resistance to infection by producing natural antibiotics.
- Reduce the duration of colds and the severity and number of symptoms.
- Decrease the frequency of chest and throat infections.
- Enhance the effect of influenza jabs.
- Lessen the severity and duration of rotavirus infections, especially in children.
- Cut the number of ear infections.
- Help the body to fight bronchitis and sinusitis.
- Reduce the risk of pneumonia.
- Lessen the need for antibiotics.

Be prepared

Hopefully, by now, you'll have introduced plenty of probiotic and prebiotic foods into your diet and may even have begun to take a regular probiotic supplement. If this is the case, your immune system should be getting a welcome boost, helping your body to become less susceptible to those annual coughs and sniffles. But if not, please do consider introducing at least some of these suggestions. Don't forget that an immune system that is primed and ready to go will respond far more quickly to serious challenges. At the very least read Chapter 9.

Below, you will find my own ideas on how to deal with colds, sore throats and other infections. These tips are based on years of experience in clinical practice and they really do seem to work. I'm not claiming cures here, but if you're quick about it and introduce them at the *first* sign of any infection, feedback strongly suggests that you can knock a cold into touch before it gets going. Don't leave it for a day, or even a few hours, to see how it develops. If possible, have the necessities to hand at home rather than wasting time going to the shops to find them. This is especially important because, once you're not feeling well, you probably won't want to go shopping. I often meet people who are streaming with a cold who tell me that they 'would have taken' the particular vitamin C or the echinacea or the probiotic that I recommended but they 'haven't had time' or they 'ran out'. The answer is to be organised and prepared. If you think this is a nuisance, consider the number of days you suffer by having to take to your bed or drag around the place feeling dreadful. If you're unlucky enough to catch the cold anyway, following the advice opposite should not only reduce discomfort but, better still, can also shorten the duration of an infection.

Action plan for colds, flu and respiratory infections

Consider the following as regular helpers:

1 Take a daily multivitamin–mineral, especially during the cold and influenza season. Studies show that multinutrient supplements taken together with probiotics for a three-month period can lessen the number and severity of symptoms and reduce the duration of a cold by several days.

2 Pick the best-quality probiotic supplement you can afford, and take it at least from October to December. Along with the other actions recommended in this chapter, doing so could lessen the risk of a cold occurring in the first place. Research results suggest that probiotics (a three-month course was followed in this particular study) can help to lessen the number of days of suffering. If cost is an issue for you in these hard times, it can still be helpful to include a daily probiotic drink or an additive-free plain yoghurt that contains live culture. Studies show that regular ingestion of probiotic bacteria helps to boost natural immunity, and although large doses may be recommended, small amounts can still be helpful.

3 Introduce Echinaforce into your daily routine throughout the winter. I use Echinaforce tincture and take 20 drops per day (in about 2.5cm/1in of water) as a maintenance dose. If I've been in close proximity to anyone who is coughing, snuffling or sneezing, I'll increase the quantity to 30 drops twice a day for at least two days. This is also the dose that I would use if I were unlucky enough to catch a cold, although since I've been taking this licensed medicine – and it's been many years now – I haven't had one.

4 Include plenty of fresh garlic in your meals whenever you can.

5 If you're going for an annual influenza jab, you might be interested to know that there's research showing that taking

189

probiotic supplements (in advance and following the injection) can enhance its effectiveness (see below).

Get fighting

If you're stricken by a bug, here's some extra support:

1 Add extra vitamin C to your daily routine. I'd take 1g (1,000mg) three times daily for seven days or until symptoms disappear. This seems like a lot, but it's very safe and extremely effective, especially when used with the supplements listed above. Buy a low-acid or buffered formula vitamin C complex (one that includes flavonoids). Try Viridian, Solgar, Bionutri or Biocare. Don't go for the plain ascorbic acid – the type that dissolves in water and is usually sold in the chemist's. It's very acidic, can upset the stomach and, in my experience, is not effective against colds.

2 Invest in a jar of Comvita Manuka Honey, which is antibacterial, anti-inflammatory and has naturally antibiotic properties, too. There are lots of different strengths, but I'd suggest trying UMF 15+. It is expensive but a worthwhile investment for medicinal purposes, stores well and lasts ages. Available from health-food stores and from www.xynergy.co.uk.

3 If you think you have an attack of full-blown influenza, probiotics may be valuable here too, whether or not you have had your annual flu jab. One study, although only small, suggested that probiotics may enhance the effectiveness of the influenza vaccine. Begin a course a couple of weeks before the injection is due and continue for two weeks following. If you're unlucky enough to be diagnosed with influenza, the herbal remedy elderberry is also excellent. Try Elderberry Complex (or Junior Elderberry) from Bionutri.

4 Check out the advice on antibiotics on page 108 and also the important hygiene advice that begins on page 118. Being scrupulous about hand washing helps enormously to reduce the spread of viruses and bacterial infections. Remember that viruses and bacteria don't just travel by air, they also spread by contact.

5 Keep fluid intake high. Drink lots of fresh juices (preferably free of sugar and additives), hot herbal tea, green tea, boiled water with fresh lime or lemon juice, sweetened with good honey (manuka if possible), mineral water, vegetable soup and chicken broth.

6 For the duration, avoid alcohol, sugar and coffee, and keep the diet light.

7 Stay at home and rest. By trying to keep going, your cold is likely to last longer and may spread to other people, who could be at greater risk of complications.

15.

Helping to Prevent
Colon Cancer

‘Ingestion of viable probiotics or prebiotics is associated with
anticarcinogenic (anti-cancer) effects. ’

Wollowski I, Rechkemmer G, Pool-Zobel BL, 'Protective Role of Probiotics
and Prebiotics in Colon Cancer', *American Journal of Clinical Nutrition*
2001;73(2 Suppl):451S–455S

At the time of writing, cancer of the colon is up there with lung,
prostate and breast cancer as one of those cancers most
frequently diagnosed. And it's getting worse. In certain parts of the
developed world, it appears poised to take over the killer top slot.

In general, cancers are usually started by some kind of alteration
(called a mutation) of a cell or by a faulty gene that kicks off
abnormal growth of cells, which then multiply and divide out of
control. Although smoking, exposure to asbestos and certain
chemicals have been identified as triggers, the causes of most
cancers remain a mystery.

When it comes to cancer of the colon, one area where we have
definite proof of something that is of real benefit in reducing risk is
making sure we eat healthily. But it looks as though there's another
helper right around the corner that could also contribute
significantly to outcome and survival. Scientific studies are focusing
more and more on the role of probiotics and prebiotics, not only as
part of a prevention package but also as possible beneficial add-ons
to existing treatments.

Looking after ourselves

Although there are some unfortunate families who are affected by a faulty gene called FAP[JB], making their susceptibility to cancer of the colon more likely, for the majority of people, the disease is considered by most health-care professionals to be almost entirely preventable. We contract colon cancer because we don't look after ourselves; in particular, we're pretty dumb about diet. We eat too much meat, load up on fat and sugar and rely on too many highly processed foods. We ignore the known health benefits of fruits, vegetables, fibre and fermented foods. We put on too much weight, take too little exercise and overdo the alcohol – then we add smoking to the list. People who abuse their bodies in this way and take the 'It'll never happen to me' attitude are all too often the ones most likely to find that it *will* happen to them!

Jargon buster

FAP stands for familial adenomatous polyposis. It's a genetic condition caused by a single faulty gene that causes multiple polyps (growths that look like cherries on stalks) to take root in the large colon. Anyone likely to inherit FAP should have very regular checkups, because this is a serious condition that can be fatal unless detected early. However, be aware that, once confirmed by a blood test and the information added to medical records, this will almost certainly affect any future applications for private medical, health or life insurance cover.

Despite the greater risk of the faulty gene being passed on through generations, thankfully it's not a foregone conclusion that the disease will occur in every offspring. Following a healthy diet rich in vegetables and fruit, and including plenty of prebiotic foods, is still important, and taking regular probiotics could be helpful.

Good gut bugs to the rescue?

You'll have seen from other parts of this book that there's a strong link between a poor diet and bungled gut bugs. So it should come as no surprise to find that there's an increasing body of research suggesting that the microflora of the bowel could have a substantial role to play in reducing the risk of a disease that is so securely linked to crappy eating habits. Adding fermented milk products, prebiotics and probiotic supplements to our regular diets could make a significant difference to our chances of avoiding cancer of the colon; for example, even a relatively small change, such as making live yoghurt a regular part of the diet, has been shown to reduce the recurrence of colonic polyps and lessen the likelihood of large bowel cancer.

What I find especially interesting is that probiotics and prebiotics – together known as synbiotics – appear to be more effective than either one or the other on their own. Researchers are looking at specific kinds of anti-cancer bacteria that they might be able to harness into therapeutic treatments and are also interested to find out whether probiotics and prebiotics could affect the genetic aspect of cancer risk. At the present time, the majority of research has been carried out in laboratories, and there needs to be many more studies involving human subjects for definite conclusions to be made. But that doesn't mean the information we have so far isn't of value:

- We already know that certain prebiotics, such as lignans (see page 96 in Chapter 6), can help to reduce the risk of cancer of the colon.

- There is also good evidence that probiotics have what are known as anti-mutagenic effects: they prevent cells from mutating and becoming cancerous. One way that they do this is to latch onto carcinogenic substances – for example, those in cooked and smoked meats – and stop them from causing damage. They also protect our internal environment from chemicals likely to cause cancer, by detoxifying any potential carcinogens that we may have swallowed. Certain types of helpful gut bugs are able to target cancer cells and deal with them so that they become harmless.

- Probiotics could offer protection against hormonal cancers, too. Beneficial bacteria are involved in the breakdown of hormones, so if our good gut bugs are depleted, unwanted oestrogens can be more easily reabsorbed into the bloodstream where they float around looking for a new home. If they find one, it's usually in a high-risk area such as breast tissue, the ovaries, prostate gland or uterus.

More help from probiotics and prebiotics

Probiotics and prebiotics may also be important in:

- Altering the ecology of the gut by controlling the bacteria that might otherwise decide to generate carcinogenic compounds.
- Producing substances that encourage programmed cell death – a process known as apoptosis. This sounds nasty but is actually helpful, because it ensures that cells that should die off do just that rather than being allowed to survive and cause trouble.
- Reducing DNA damage caused by chemical carcinogens to certain types of cell in the colon.
- Binding and degrading potential cancer-causing substances, such as nitrosamines.
- Lowering the acid balance (pH) of the colon, which discourages the growth of pathogens that might become tumour promoters.
- Stimulating the immune system (see page 255) to be more efficient at defending the body against cancer cells by producing those important anti-tumour and anti-mutagenic compounds so that the body can better protect itself against invaders.

Action plan for reducing your risk

Most risk reduction comes down to common-sense eating. Here are my ten top essentials:

1 **Read** and act upon the information in the section on constipation coming up on page 199.

2 Remember that dietary fibre is an essential for anyone serious about improving their chances of avoiding this disease. Chapter 6 on fibre and Chapter 4 on prebiotics are essential reading.

3 Drink more water. Most people don't take enough fluid and this has a direct effect on bowel health. Getting through 1.5 litres ($2^3/_4$ pints) of water per day in addition to tea and juice, is believed to significantly reduce the risk of cancer of the bladder, breast and colon.

4 Cut back on red meat (and especially burgers, smoked and preserved meats, and pork products, which includes sausages, bacon and ham). Meat eaters seem to be more prone to this type of cancer than those who eat little or no red meat. One of the reasons may be that when meat proteins are broken down, they produce toxins and carcinogenic substances. In small amounts, the body copes, but where there is a high red-meat consumption, the colon can get swamped. Good gut flora, particularly when taken in conjunction with foods that are rich in prebiotic fibre, are believed to be protective and to reduce and deactivate toxic compounds.

5 Eat more fresh fish and white meat, but have a go at some vegetarian dishes, too. No, I'm not talking about a life of lettuce and lentils. Forget cranky and think scrumptious. There are lots of fabulous food ideas that don't involve meat. Most vegetarian recipes are not only rich in prebiotic fibre, vitamins and minerals but they're also filling, satisfying and lots cheaper to put together than meals of animal protein. So think of all the money you'll save. And vegetarian meals can be really easy to make; great if you're on a time treadmill or you think you can't cook. Beans are especially good and have excellent fibre scores. At least once a week during the winter I make a bean curry with mild spices, garlic, onions, tomatoes, carrots, potatoes and all kinds of pulses, including red kidney beans, haricot beans, butter beans, chickpeas and lentils. Just fry the onion and the garlic in the spices, throw in the chopped vegetables and the beans (for convenience use canned or bottled beans, not dried, and make sure to rinse off the canning or bottling water before use). Add a glass of red wine, a quarter teaspoon of salt and a can of chopped tomatoes, then simmer for an hour. It's cooked when the carrots are tender. Serve with brown basmati rice or couscous.

6 Check pack labels and avoid processed and manufactured low-fat foods that contain artificial additives and fat substitutes.

7 Include plain yoghurts that contain live cultures. It might also be worthwhile taking a probiotic drink every day. Studies show that *Lactobacillus casei Shirota* lessened the recurrence of colonic polyps which can be a precursor to colon cancer.

8 Up your intake of fresh fruit, vegetables and salad foods. Most are not only an excellent source of additional fibre but are also rich in antioxidants, which already have a terrific anti-cancer track record.

9 Find out what a unit of alcohol really looks like, and then be honest with yourself about intake. Don't forget that the official recommendations are maximum figures, not minimum.

10 Give up smoking. It is devastating to the digestive system. It's long been associated with lung cancer, but it's now known that smokers are also putting themselves nearer the front of the queue for colon cancer, too. It's a terrible way to die.

Be body aware

If you notice any changes in bowel habit, any bleeding, dark colour or black in your stools, constipation of more than a couple of days, sudden diarrhoea with no obvious cause, pain, discomfort or distension that won't go away, then **see your doctor without delay**. If diagnosed in the early stages, this cancer is one of the easiest to treat successfully. If there's a screening programme for your age group in your area, get yourself on to it.

No magic bullets

The information I've referred to in this chapter should be looked upon as good prevention. I'm not suggesting for a moment that diet or supplements can cure cancer. Nor is it a question of simply relying on a probiotic pill and expecting it to work in the presence of rubbish food, booze and cigarettes. But taking all these things together, it certainly looks as though probiotics and prebiotics might have an important influence on our intestines, which could significantly reduce the risk of contracting cancer of the colon or rectum, and perhaps other types of cancer, too. It's worth considering, don't you think?

16.

How Often Do You Open Your Bowels?

If you're a 'go once a day, regular as clockwork' type of person, you might be pleasantly satisfied with your routine and consider yourself to be healthy as far as your own personal refuse department is concerned. Once a day is what most medical experts accept as normal, although some disagree and say it isn't often enough. It's certainly always been my view that twice or even three times a day is much more healthy than a single visit.

In terms of evolution, it certainly seems that going only once a day could be bordering on being constipated. Although our diets and our food supply have both evolved and changed beyond all recognition over the last few hundred years, and markedly so since the 1950s, the human digestive system hasn't. It's all been a bit of a shock for the poor old intestines, which are nevertheless expected to deal with a hugely complex mix of modern-day foods, many of them heavily processed, highly refined and loaded with artificial additives that have only been around for the blink of an eye. We just assume that the old gut will get on with the job and not grumble. But how can it digest, absorb or eliminate efficiently if we don't give it the right kind of fuel? Would you put the wrong petrol in your car?

In the days when we were cave dwellers or hunter-gatherers, our food intake was generally much more fibrous and, as a consequence, our bowels much more active. Once for every meal was more likely the norm than the once a week suffered by some people today. Although you might be surprised, I have seen patients who think once a fortnight is frequent!

Any single visit where you find that you need to sit for ages or your bowels don't respond unless you push or strain, almost certainly suggests that you're bunged up. This is no joke. Clogged and compacted colons have long been associated with an increased risk of diverticular disease, haemorrhoids and colon cancer. Speeding up the elimination of dietary leftovers is more than common sense. It should be considered as vital preventative medicine.

Bad bathroom habits

It's interesting to see how familiar routines can be so hard to break. I've had some patients – especially those with conditions such as diverticular disease or chronic constipation, thoroughly settled into a pattern of emptying their bowels a couple of times a week – who are horrified by the change. Despite the fact that they're going properly for the first time for years, perhaps in their entire lives, at first they worry that this is abnormal. It isn't. I've even had some people protest that they had 'diarrhoea' when it turned out to be just two visits to pass simple, well-formed stools. One lady actually complained that she would have to curtail her new high-fibre diet because it was (and I quote) 'making me go to the toilet' and that this was 'inconvenient'. It took me a long time to persuade her that the 'inconvenience' might be the thing that saved her from colon cancer.

> ### Talking of bowel movements ...
> Those of you who are regular readers of my jottings will already know that I suffer from a morbid interest in the colour, consistency and odour of excreta and am a firm believer that we should all check the paper or the pan at least once a week so that we're aware of what our own wastes actually look like. They're a really important indicator of how healthy you are – or not! The section on poo colours (page 204) is helpful and fun. There's also a no-holds-barred discussion about bowel movements in my book *Good Gut Healing*. And for anyone who feels the urge to find out more about the impact and importance of waste products, do have a look at a wonderful website called www.blueherbs.co.uk/articles/colon_cleansing_poo.asp and enjoy their Poo Contest. But be warned, this is defecatingly *not* one for the squeamish!

As part of my regular clinic work, I give dietary advice to help reduce the risk of constipation and the problems associated with it. Even in today's supposed enlightenment and free expression, I'm amazed and distressed at how often a patient will say that they've had the symptoms for weeks or months but were too embarrassed, or too busy, to visit the doctor. Nothing sexist intended here, but it's nearly always men who procrastinate.

Rest assured that your doctor won't be embarrassed

Can I remind you of something else you probably already know but don't think about too often? Your GP has likely seen more backsides and done more examinations of them than you could possibly imagine. So if you're worried, ask for help and don't be shy. The good doctor will always prefer that you bothered him or her and had your mind put at rest rather than be faced with the distress of having to tell you that you have bowel cancer. As one doctor friend of mine likes to say, 'Better the collywobbles than cancer.'

What can you do to make a difference?

When constipation strikes, one of the first things we may think of is a laxative. The occasional use of a laxative should be no problem, but if you find you're needing to use over-the-counter products on a frequent basis, then something isn't right. What you should really be paying attention to is (1) the state of your gut flora; (2) how much fluid you're taking in; and (3) how much and what kind of dietary fibre you're using.

1 A sluggish bowel is often the result of disturbed intestinal bacteria: that is not having enough good gut bugs. I always use some kind of probiotic supplement as part of the treatment for constipation. The results can be remarkable. There's good evidence from scientific studies that improving the diet and adding the right probiotic bacteria is a healthy recipe for

preventing and treating what doctors call 'slow transit'. Certainly probiotics have the ability to stimulate a sluggish colon and to shift stagnant faeces, especially when used in conjunction with plenty of prebiotic foods and a monitored increase in fluid intake.

2 I would also say that the vast majority of patients who complain about infrequent visits to the toilet don't drink enough water. One of the causes of dry, hard and stagnant or slow-moving faeces can be inadequate fluid.

3 Worryingly high numbers of people have far too little fibre in their diets, but there are also folks who eat significant quantities of high-fibre bran every day and still find they struggle to pass a daily motion. Increasing our intake of roughage, we're told by advertisers of nosebag breakfast cereals, will make us 'regular'! Well, yes, but there's far more to a healthy colon than spooning string and sawdust into your mouth every morning. Be comforted that there are other types of fibre which have a much more effective action and are a lot kinder to the gut.

These three points above are all interlinked, vitally supporting one another. To maintain a well-behaved bowel, it's vital to drink plenty of fluid, which then acts with the fibre to keep the wastes moving, and also helps to create a suitable terrain for good gut bugs to thrive.

Promise me that you'll see your doctor if:

- You're constipated and have been so for more than a few days.
- Your constipation is worsening despite all your best efforts.
- Your bowel habits have changed in any way without obvious reason.
- You spend a long time sitting before anything happens or you have to strain.
- You rarely manage a bowel movement unless you use a laxative.
- You don't open your bowels very often but seem to be constantly emptying your bladder (being constipated can mean that you urinate more frequently because of the pressure of the colon against the bladder).

- You have uncontrolled leakage of faeces or repeated attacks of underwear-destroying wet wind (this can happen even if you are constipated).

- You suffer any kind of pain or nausea when you try to go to the toilet.

- Your faeces are what could be considered 'permanent floaters' that bounce like corks and resist the flush (it could be that you are not absorbing fats and oils from your diet, a serious condition which needs immediate investigation).

- Your faeces are small in size and quantity, dry and shaped like pebbles or mini cannonballs or peas (consider all of these as constipated stools). Long thin strings – especially if they are becoming progressively narrower over time – can indicate colon or rectal cancer.

- You feel as if you're passing broken glass (could be haemorrhoids or an anal fissure).

- Your wastes are persistently really foul smelling. I don't mean just a bit more odorous than usual, but room-emptyingly unpleasant all the time. (This could be caused by a number of different problems but will almost always involve a large bowel that doesn't have enough good bacteria – don't forget that bad bugs hum.)

- You pass anything that resembles bits of white string or thin spaghetti (both indicate the presence of parasites).

- You're suffering loose stools to the point of diarrhoea on some days and chronic constipation on others.

- You see any blood mixed with your stools. If the blood is dark red or faeces appear to be streaked with black, see your doctor without delay. The same applies if the pan water is bloody. While bright red blood can be a sign of a pile (haemorrhoids) or an anal fissure, dark or black blood in the stools could indicate that there is bleeding further up inside the digestive tract, possibly in the stomach. Whatever the cause, continued bleeding can lead not only to anaemia but could indicate a serious illness that requires immediate attention.

When you see the doctor, don't forget to say:

- How long the constipation has been a problem.
- How often you go to the toilet.
- Which remedies you have tried.
- Whether your faeces are hard, soft or mucusy.
- If there is a history of constipation in your family.
- If there is a history of bowel cancer.

There's a lot more detailed advice about how to deal with constipation in my book *Good Gut Healing*. In the meantime, because having the courage to examine your own waste products could save your life, here's a reminder of the 'colour chart' that comes from that book.

Shades of s**t

Different foods can have a fairly immediate effect on the tone, tint or intensity of excreta, so being aware of what you've eaten in the last 24 hours is a good way to avoid unnecessary concern that something is wrong. An occasional difference is more than likely nothing to worry about, but if the colour alters significantly and stays that way for more than a couple of days, I would definitely suggest a visit to see your doctor or practice nurse.

All tones of red and black

- Some iron supplements, especially prescription ones, which can be constipating in their own right, are likely to make waste products appear dark, possibly even black. That's because this type of iron is not well absorbed with the result that much of it ends up in the large intestine instead of where it's supposed to be: in the bloodstream.
- Medications that contain bismuth (sometimes used in the treatment of digestive ulcers and as an ingredient in antacid preparations) can result in much darker stools.

- If you've eaten any sweets containing liquorice, you should know that this can add black patches to your poo.

- Dark red berry fruits such as those found in 'black forest' mixtures, could even make it a bit purple. And so could beetroot.

- Chewed up tomato skin may also pass through undigested in some people and at first glance can look uncomfortably like splatters of blood.

Alert:

- Bright red blood on the paper is more than likely going to be due to a haemorrhoid or an anal fissure or split, and although they can lead to complications if they're not treated as soon as possible, they're not life threatening. Haemorrhoids (piles) are often associated with or caused by constipation, in which case the information I've already given you on the previous page applies.

- Stools that appear to be totally black, striped or very dark can be caused by a bleeding ulcer or other internal bleeding.

- If you see dark red on the paper or the pan, this suggests there may be bleeding in the large intestine. It could be an early indication of colon cancer and requires *immediate* medical advice and investigation. And I mean *immediate*.

Orange/green/yellow

- If you're taking a multivitamin supplement that contains ribo-flavin, otherwise known as vitamin B_2, bear in mind that its natural colour is orange and that it can create an interesting orangey green pigment to your daily doings. It can certainly give a dramatic dayglo to your urine. Don't worry; it's harmless and beneficial.

- Another cause of yellow, yellowy brown or green could simply be the result of yesterday's meal, especially if it contained a lot of carrots, spinach, pumpkin squash, curry or other spices, especially turmeric.

- Sweetcorn, being wickedly fibrous, will often pass through without even changing its shape, so if you've been supping sweetcorn chowder or nibbling at corn on the cob, don't be surprised to see your dodies dotted with yellow.

Alert:

- The same yellow/green hue could also signal problems in the gallbladder or liver. Or it could be a side effect of some types of antibiotic. And, of course, it's the colour we know so well if we're stricken with what is affectionately called 'the squits' or 'the runs', otherwise known as infectious diarrhoea.

Grey or cream

Alert:

- Pale grey or porridge-coloured wastes could mean more serious problems to do with the pancreas, malabsorption of fats, or something wrong with the gallbladder or a blocked bile duct. However, eating porridge is good for your intestines and does not make faeces porridge coloured.

- Mucus or pus in the stools are common in irritable bowel syndrome, diverticular disease and inflammatory bowel disease, but even more seriously can be associated with gastrointestinal cancer, in particular of the stomach or colon.

Boring brown is best

The healthiest hue is said to be a kind of medium brown with an easy consistency that doesn't require any straining. Fluffy round the edges is also good.

Sticky and stuck or soft and slippery?

You might be interested to know that high-fibre stools are two to three times as bulky as those lacking fibre. By adding bulk to the diet, more fluid is absorbed – rather like taking a dry sponge and pushing it down into a bowl of water. Once soaked, wastes are softer, 'cleaner' (less mucusy), more pliable and easier to pass. And transit time is speeded up from a sluggish 36 hours or more to somewhere between 12 and 24 hours. As a result, the gut is healthier, because wastes don't get a chance to hang around and go off. In fact, fibre actually helps to clean up the encrusted walls and stimulate local circulation. Although a large proportion of the water content is reabsorbed as the faeces work their way through each section of the large intestine, sufficient moisture should remain at the end of the passageway to make for comfortable defecation.

Low-fibre diets, on the other hand, make for tacky, mucus-laden faeces that stick to the colon wall. This allows abnormal bacteria to build up, producing potentially harmful carcinogenic substances. Elimination can be slow and poor, taking three times as long – or longer – to make the journey. Dry, dense stools need much greater pressure and force to reach the exit. And it puts undue strain on the colon walls. Some wastes shun daylight altogether and never reach the outside world at all, jamming themselves up against the wall and sticking to side pouches where they putrefy (go off), then solidify and stick.

Don't let this happen to you.

Action plan for relieving constipation

Keep your bowels healthy by following the suggestions below:

1 **Allow yourself undisturbed time** to visit the bathroom, and never ignore the urge to go. But never strain. Allow things to happen naturally. If they don't, then take the following steps:

2 **Check out your existing diet** by referring to the Swaps on page 50 and think seriously about treating yourself to a Good Gut Upgrade (Chapter 2). In particular, don't rely on breakfast bran as your major source of roughage, especially if you have any kind of bowel problem. Include a variety of different types of dietary fibre. Read Chapter 6, Fabulous Fibre, and Chapter 4, Prebiotics – Your Probiotic Support Group.

3 **Up your intake of fluid.** Drink more water, fresh juices, green and black tea, herbal teas and soups.

4 **Add live yoghurt**, probiotic shots, buttermilk or kefir to your daily diet.

5 **Up your intake of dietary fibre**. See Chapter 6 on Fabulous Fibre.

6 Consider regular colon cleansing. There are several different herbal packs available. You might try a simple fibre detox or a more in-depth herbal colon cleanse.

7 Get moving. Regular exercise isn't only good for your heart, it exercises your insides too.

8 Massage your abdomen every day. Use about half a tea-spoonful of extra virgin olive oil and massage in a circular action over the whole of the belly area. Not only does this help to move faeces along your internal tubing but it also releases gas, so unless you are in a comfortable long-term relationship with a significant other, then it's probably best done in private.

9 Learn to relax and let go. Don't be a constipated personality.

10 Join the probiotics movement. Follow a course of best-quality probiotic supplements – certainly until the constipation is re-solved and, if possible, continue for two to three months. Then repeat the same course for a month every few months (see Chapter 25).

11 Don't forget to see your doctor if you are persistently constipated, are in pain or you notice any changes in bowel habit.

A note about irritable bowel syndrome

Much of the advice in the above section is also helpful for IBS. More information on this condition follows on in Chapter 18.

17.

Dealing with Diarrhoea

‘For more than 100 years, probiotic remedies . . . have been used to fight infection. Now, substantial scientific and clinical evidence indicates that certain well-selected [probiotics] can reduce the risk and duration of diarrhea. ’

Dr Gregor Reid, 'Probiotics in the Treatment of Diarrheal Diseases',
Current Infectious Disease Reports 2000;2(1):78

Of all the research carried out using probiotics, the condition that has probably been investigated in the greatest detail is the prevention and treatment of diarrhoea.

Probiotics have already proven themselves to be a safe remedy for both infectious and antibiotic-related diarrhoea in premature babies, toddlers and children, and in adults too, especially for the elderly, for people suffering or recovering from food poisoning and for traveller's diarrhoea. Probiotics are also being looked at in connection with the prevention and treatment of rotavirus, a really nasty virus that causes gastroenteritis and diarrhoea that, at its worst, can be fatal (it results in nearly one million deaths worldwide each year).

Studies show repeatedly that probiotics, in the form of drinks and as supplements, can help people stricken with diarrhoea caused by the superbug *Clostridium difficile*. Probiotics may further help as a preventive, to reduce the spread of the disease: it's been demonstrated that patients who were given twice-daily probiotic drinks not only had far less incidence of diarrhoea but they also had none of the dangerous bacteria showing up in their waste products.

Did you know?

The usual definition for diarrhoea is having several urgent liquid or near-liquid bowel movements per 24 hours. If you have three normal bowel movements a day, it doesn't mean that you have diarrhoea.

There are very many different types of diarrhoeal illness, but the most common causes of diarrhoea include:

- Side effects of antibiotics.
- Hospital-borne bacterial infections.
- Contaminated food or water.

Cryptosporidium (found in infected water), *Salmonella*, *Campylobacter*, *Listeria* and certain types of *E. coli* are some of the main bacterial sources of diarrhoea.

Not only can probiotics be extremely helpful at easing the symptoms of diarrhoea and speeding recovery but they're also considered a valuable preventive. People who take regular probiotic foods or supplements seem to be at less risk of contracting bacterial infections and, if they take them alongside any essential antibiotic treatment, there are fewer side effects.

Note: the probiotic yeast known as *Saccharomyces boulardii* has been found in several different studies to be helpful against diarrhoea caused by antibiotics, *Clostridium difficile*, contaminated food, and in the treatment of infectious diarrhoea, which can be triggered by the really nasty 'tummy bug', *Campylobacter*. However, this particular probiotic supplement should not be used without medical supervision, as it may be unsuitable for some conditions.

Take care

Keep in mind that diarrhoea in babies and young children can be very serious, possibly life-threatening. If symptoms persist for more than 12 hours in newborns or 24 hours in toddlers, get medical advice first from your local GP. If he or she is not available, contact NHS Direct or your nearest A&E.

Action plan against diarrhoea

To avoid and treat diarrhoea, follow the suggestions below:

1 **Follow the advice on hygiene** and how to reduce the risk of bacterial resistance in Chapter 7.

2 **If you're taking any kind of acid-suppressing medication**, perhaps for conditions such as reflux or hiatus hernia, don't use it long term unless you're seeing your doctor for regular checkups and discussion. These medicines work by knocking out stomach acid, which, of course, can be extremely helpful if excess hydrochloric acid (HCl) is causing you problems. However, HCl is one of our first lines of defence against bacteria, which means that without it we are more susceptible to the types of bacteria that can result in diarrhoeal illness. Overuse of such drugs, especially those known as proton pump inhibitors (check your prescription leaflet) are associated with an increased risk of contracting the superbug *Clostridium difficile* and have been blamed for masking symptoms of the ulcer bacteria *Helicobacter pylori*.

3 **Probiotics could prevent a holiday being ruined by diarrhoea**. People from developed countries who visit tropical or sub-tropical zones are three times more likely than the hardier locals to go down with traveller's tum. And although most of us are savvy enough to be cautious about what we eat when we're away, especially if we're off to far-flung shores where water or food supplies might be suspect, any extra help is always welcome.

It's interesting that researchers have made particular note that the benefit depends on consistent use of the product and that larger doses were more effective. It's for this reason that I usually advise doubling the recommended dose for the duration of the overseas visit. You might also invest in one of the hygiene packs designed for hospital patients, which are also extremely useful on holiday.

Top travel tip

If you're going on a flight anywhere, take Dr Vogel's Echinaforce tincture twice a day together with a top-quality probiotic for at least one week before travel. Continue while you're away and for a further week on your return. Some good probiotic brands don't require refrigeration and are ideal for taking with you.

If you've been around someone who has a bug, follow the same advice, but continue the course for a further five days after symptoms have subsided.

Remember that by reducing the risk of getting an infection, you also reduce the likelihood of needing to take antibiotics.

4 Include probiotic yoghurts and shots regularly in your diet, and twice daily if you're waiting to go into hospital or are there already. Talk with your doctor or consultant about a course of probiotic supplements. The more consistent and longer the intake, the better the protection is likely to be.

5 Whatever the type or possible cause of your diarrhoea, follow the all-important rule of keeping your fluid intake high. Avoid coffee, strong tea, alcohol and carbonated drinks. Stick to plain mineral or filtered water and herbal teas, and use rehydration drinks to replace fluids and essential minerals. Remember that fruit juices, especially apple juice, can aggravate diarrhoea in some people and are, in any event, best diluted 50:50 with water. If you feel like eating, keep the diet light. Plain boiled brown rice and plain additive-free full-fat yoghurt may sound boring but are two of the best foods to help settle a raging stomach or explosive bowel.

6 If the situation has not resolved within 36 hours, see your doctor.

18.

Irritable Bowel Syndrome

Of all the conditions that I see in clinic, the one that seems to be the most persistently misunderstood is irritable bowel syndrome (IBS). Symptoms generally follow a pattern of long periods of constipation interspersed with episodes of urgent diarrhoea and accompanied by abdominal pain, bloating and excessive wind. There is very often a sensitivity or intolerance to one or more foods, usually including wheat and/or dairy. The problem for the doctor trying to make a sound diagnosis is that tests are rarely helpful. Perhaps this absence of physical proof is the reason why IBS used to be dismissed as being 'all in the mind' or treated as a psychological disorder.

It's worth highlighting the sad fact that IBS has long been – and unfortunately remains – a bit of a cop-out conclusion for almost any gut symptoms that have no other explanation, with the result that a lot of people think they have – or are told they have – IBS when they don't. However, I do also see patients who have serious, full-scale IBS and it is to such people that this chapter is directed. I hope its contents will help you.

The bad news

Although investigations into the causes of irritable bowel syndrome are ongoing and no one has yet come up with a conclusive set of parameters, it looks as though disturbed gut flora might, at least, be one of the triggers even if it's not the only culprit.

Interestingly, IBS often follows a bout of gastroenteritis or food poisoning, or a gut infection that has been treated with antibiotics. The condition has also been linked to something called SIBO – small intestinal bacterial overgrowth[JB]. Studies show that probiotics can improve the symptoms of SIBO and reduce its toxic effects.

> **Jargon buster**
>
> **SIBO** (small intestinal bacterial overgrowth) is a condition where the number of bacteria in the small intestine increase above normal. No one knows for sure why it happens in some people. It may be more common where the ileocaecal valve – the junction between your small and large intestines – is slack and allows wastes to flow back up the pipe bringing unwanted bacteria along with it. Patients on kidney dialysis or who are suffering with hypochlorhydria (low levels of stomach acid) or IBS can also be affected.

The food sensitivity aspect of IBS is believed to be caused by an out-of-order fermentation process. This is where food leftovers in the intestines aren't broken down fully, leading to an excess of foaming, farting and bloating – disturbance which has been linked to low levels of normal friendly flora such as *Bifidobacteria* and *Lactobacilli*. Lack of protection from helpful flora can affect the permeability of the gut wall, which then allows bad bacteria to sneak into the gut lining or even climb through to the bloodstream itself (see leaky gut syndrome on page 244).

IBS has been further associated with unwelcome gut parasites, malabsorption of fructose – a natural sugar found in many foods – and with immune disorders such as fibromyalgia and IBD (inflammatory bowel disease). Although IBS and IBD are not the same thing, researchers have even wondered if, in some cases, IBS might be mistaken for early signs of coeliac disease, Crohn's disease or ulcerative colitis.

The good news

Studies suggest that probiotics might strengthen the barrier between the gut and the bloodstream, restoring normal function, so reducing the risk of leaky gut syndrome and allergic reactions. There is also promising evidence that probiotics ease abdominal cramps, bloating, gas and inflammation, improve stool consistency, lessen pain and gas, and help the movement of the gut, thereby reducing the number of urgent bathroom visits.

Case history

A lady aged 38 was referred to me with IBS. She had been diagnosed at 18 and, to use her own words was 'told to eat more bran and get on with it'. In the intervening 20 years, she had suffered constant abdominal pain and bloating, but no other IBS symptoms. This is a very common scenario and one that I have seen many times. Following an intensive investigation into her diet, I recommended that she exclude all wheat products, especially bread and bran cereal, introduce milled flax, eat plain live yoghurt for breakfast, drink more water and take a three-month course of probiotics, repeated every six months, to ensure that healthy gut flora levels were maintained. In less than four weeks all the symptoms disappeared and, most importantly, she has had no more pain. She tells me that she feels completely well for the first time in her adult life.

Action plan for IBS

Help IBS symptoms by following the suggestions below:

1 Avoid these foods and ingredients: beer and spirits, corn (maize), cow's milk, fructose, soft drinks, sorbitol, sugar and foods that contain sugar, sweet wines and sherry, wheat, especially bread and breakfast bran, yeast, artificial flavourings.

2 Take great care to check all food labels for hidden troublemakers. Wheat flour, modified starch, maize, yeast, sugar, sorbitol and fructose are often used as additives, and all can be IBS aggravators! So too can sugar, which is added to savoury as well as sweet foods and sometimes used as a base ingredient in flavourings. Be aware that sorbitol, found in many diabetic foods and in some medicines and sweets can cause diarrhoea if eaten too often. Lots of prescription and over-the-counter preparations contain sweeteners, artificial colours and flavours.

3 Treat sweetened probiotic drinks with caution unless and until you are happy that they are not aggravating your condition. Most contain added sugars and many are cow's milk based. Plain sheep's milk or goat's milk yoghurt may be a better option. You could also try kefir or buttermilk.

4 Don't ever be persuaded that bran flakes or any other kind of wheat-bran cereal is helpful for IBS, even if it is recommended by your doctor. Apologies to any doctors reading this but wheat products nearly always make matters much worse. Use the dietary fibre and prebiotic food lists on pages 85 and 103 instead.

5 Introduce small amounts of milled flax fibre or psyllium husk fibre into your diet. Page 95 has details.

6 Chew every mouthful thoroughly. This really helps a sensitive gut to cope more easily.

7 Remember that cooked vegetables may suit you better than raw. Cooking breaks down the fibre content and loses some of the fructose, the natural sugar content of the food.

8 Keep a food diary and see if there is any relationship between your diet and the pattern of IBS flare-ups.

9 If the situation doesn't improve, ask to be tested for fructose allergy. It can be done with a simple breath test. The problem seems to be that if fructose doesn't get digested and passes in its raw state into the large bowel, bacteria feast on it and, as we saw in Chapter 10 on dysbiosis, create all sorts of problems, including diarrhoea, bloating and flatulence. It's when gas seeps into the bloodstream that it can be detected in the breath. If your doctor isn't familiar with the procedure, ask for a referral to a specialist who genuinely understands the condition (unfortunately, many do not).

10 Incorporate plenty of foods from the prebiotic list on page 85. Prebiotic foods used in conjunction with probiotics may be one of the best ways of dealing with IBS symptoms.

11 Take a regular probiotic supplement. You may need to try more than one brand before finding the one that helps you best, because IBS is a very individual condition, and what suits one person may not work for another. In my own work with IBS patients, I have found *Lactobacillus acidophilus* helpful in some cases but generally not nearly as effective as *Bifidobacterium infantis*. There are some scientific studies that support this view. *B. infantis* is sometimes sold as a supplement for babies. (Supplier info in Resources.) If your symptoms were triggered by an infection such as *Campylobacter enteritis*, research results suggest that it may be wise to take a combination product containing several different strains of probiotics for several months in order to fully restore your good gut bugs.

12 Avoid FOS (fructo-oligosaccharides). Although often extremely helpful for many conditions, FOS may not be suitable for people suffering IBS because of the common problem of fructose malabsorption. However, acacia bark (see page 76) is a good alternative.

19.

Good Gut Flora and Lactose Intolerance

Lactose is the name we give to the natural sugar content of cow's milk. Lactase is the enzyme that we need in our bodies to digest that milk sugar. Lactose intolerance is the condition we get if we have a deficiency of the lactase enzyme and yet still drink milk. The condition may be inherited, in which case it's known as primary intolerance. Or it can be 'acquired' which means that the problem is the result of a digestive disorder, an infection, stomach surgery or the simple process of ageing. Humans are more tolerant of milk sugar in the early years of life when it's vital to absorb as much nourishment as possible from a mother's milk, but just because we take it as babies, doesn't necessarily mean it's easily digested in adults. Generally, the older we get the less lactase we produce and so, potentially, the more lactose intolerant we become.

Lactic-acid bacteria are certain types of friendly flora that can convert undigested lactose into lactic acid, thereby making the milk sugar less of a problem. Including strains such as *Lactobacillus acidophilus*, *Lactobacillus bulgaricus* and *Streptococcus thermophilus* in our regular diet is known to help lactose-intolerant people digest milk products more fully. This doesn't mean, however, that probiotics can cure lactose intolerance, merely that they assist digestion and prevent some symptoms.

What's normal?

Lactose intolerance is incredibly common. In fact, the condition is so widespread that it would be fairer to say that lactose intolerance is the norm and lactose tolerance the rarer condition. In many countries around the globe the pasteurised milk products that we so favour in northern Europe and North America are simply not part of the natural staple diet. It's been estimated that between two-thirds and three-quarters of the world's population, including most Asian, Arab, African, Mediterranean, Jewish and Oriental peoples, are not able to digest cow's milk efficiently simply because their bodies are not programmed to manufacture the necessary enzyme. The reason that Northern Europeans were, certainly in the past, more likely to be able to cope with milk is an evolutionary thing. In countries with low levels of sunshine, milk would have been a vital source of nourishment, in particular for vitamin D. There is evidence that Iron Age man in Scotland drank milk (although perhaps more likely from sheep or goat rather than cow).

What happens inside?

When milk sugar passes through the digestive system without being digested, it'll end up in the large intestine where it's probably going to be pounced on by a whole load of moody microbes looking for a methane fix. One way or the other, the result is gas, bloating, abdominal discomfort and loose, watery waste products.

Healthier options?

If any of the above symptoms plague you when you drink milk, of course it's certainly worth adding probiotics to the diet to see if they will help. Although one study found that mixing probiotics with cow's milk-based infant formula made no difference, there's good evidence from other studies and also from clinical experience that supplementing beneficial bacteria can help reduce symptoms of milk allergies.

Cow's milk products, when properly digested, are an important source of calcium and other nutrients. Some cheeses and yoghurts made from cow's milk may be better digested than cow's milk itself because the lactose is partially or totally broken down during the manufacturing process. However, this most mucus-forming of foods can still cause a range of other problems aside from lactose intolerance, including aggravation of eczema, asthma, catarrh and sinusitis. Don't worry; if you're a sufferer of one or more of these symptoms, there are better alternatives available.

It's well documented that lactose-intolerant individuals cope better with fermented dairy products, such as yoghurt, kefir and buttermilk and suffer far fewer symptoms than if they consume similar quantities of ordinary milk. The bacteria which are used as starter cultures for yoghurt products produce their own lactase during the fermentation process, making the yoghurt easier to digest and therefore potentially more nourishing than straight cow's milk. You might also try sheep's or goat's milk yoghurts and cheeses which, patient experience suggests, are often more suitable than their cow's milk equivalents, being less inclined to cause discomfort simply because they're better digested.

Something else to bear in mind is that you might still be what is known as a maldigester of milk without being lactose intolerant. It's also possible to be hypersensitive even if you have the lactase enzyme. Studies suggest that even in people who are mildly hypersensitive to milk and milk products, the addition of probiotic foods to the diet can reduce the associated inflammation.

20.

The Ulcer Bug: *Helicobacter Pylori*

❝In the group taking probiotic yogurt alongside antibiotic therapy, side effects were fewer and the rate of eradication of *Helicobacter pylori* significantly higher than in those following the medication therapy only. ❞

H.B. Yang, et al., 'Pretreatment with *Lactobacillus-* and *Bifidobacterium-* containing yogurt can improve the efficacy of quadruple therapy in eradicating residual *Helicobacter pylori* infection after failed triple therapy', *American Journal of Clinical Nutrition* 2006;83:864–9

Most people are aware by now that the majority of digestive ulcers are caused by a bacterium called *Helicobacter pylori*. Usually associated with the stomach, it can also set up home in the lower part of the gullet as well as the upper part of the small intestine (the duodenum). It does its dirty work by causing inflammation (gastritis), which upsets the mechanisms that control acid production and, if left untreated, can lead to gastric cancer.

What is not always realised is that, although the infection is commonly associated with excess acidity, it can also colonise the stomachs of people who already suffer with low levels of acid. In fact, although *Helicobacter* is usually talked about in terms of an overproduction of gastric acid, it doesn't actually like acidic conditions and hides from them by sneaking into the protective layer of mucus and skin cells that line the stomach and digestive tract.

The accepted method of dealing with a *Helicobacter* infection is one week of a medical combination known as triple therapy, which includes two different kinds of antibiotic plus a third drug, usually

> ## Very important point
> It's worth mentioning here that *H. pylori* happily hangs around the stomachs of approximately half the population, and yet only around 10 per cent of these go on to have problems. It's perfectly possible to be a carrier with no symptoms and yet still pass the bug on to other people who are more susceptible to recurring infections. I've seen several cases where patients have been treated successfully for the ulcer but then suffered repeated bouts of reinfection. After some investigations, the source of the new infection was found to be the patient's spouse. If you have had more than one episode of the ulcer bug, then it's worth asking your doctor to screen other members of the family. Researchers think that diet and lifestyle also play a significant role in whether or not the disease develops.

a proton pump inhibitor or similar, designed to suppress stomach acid. Treatment is usually, although not always, successful (occasionally quadruple therapy is necessary) but, as with anything that requires antibiotics, there is always the problem of side effects and of damage to the natural gut flora.

Probiotic support

The results of studies that have looked at probiotics as part and parcel of the treatment for *H. pylori* have been mixed but are generally very positive and show that certain strains of lactic acid bacteria, such as *Lactobacillus acidophilus*, can hold back *Helicobacter*, creating conditions that will inhibit its growth, deter it from attaching itself to the gut wall and, at the same time, calm the associated inflammation. Probiotics have also been shown to decrease the activity of a particular enzyme, called urease, which *H. pylori* bugs need in order to survive in the acidic stomach.

There's good evidence, too, that it's beneficial to take probiotics at the same time as standard ulcer management. Probiotic supplements are shown to prevent or reduce the side effects of *H. pylori* treatment and have made patients more comfortable so that they were more inclined to complete the all-important triple therapy. Regular use of fermented milk products may also be valuable in controlling the bacteria.

Action plan for *Helicobacter pylori*

Help rid yourself of *Helicobacter pylori* by following the suggestions below:

1 Ask for proper tests to be carried out before accepting antibiotic treatment. A breath test (known as a urea test) will tell you if *H. pylori* is present now, whereas a blood test can reveal if it has been around in the past.

2 If symptoms persist after treatment, go back to your doctor for further checks. Remember that the accepted method of dealing with a *Helicobacter* infection is an antibiotic combo that includes two different kinds of antibiotic, so if you are prescribed only one type of antibiotic for this condition, it's absolutely vital that you ask why. It's becoming all too common for patients to be refused triple therapy on the basis that it's too expensive. I've seen several people (all UK based) who had been diagnosed with *H. pylori* and were prescribed only one antibiotic. Not surprisingly, it didn't work. In each case, triple therapy was considered a last resort so, in fact, the cost (and potential risk to the patient of not being properly treated) was actually greater overall.

3 If you're affected repeatedly by *H. pylori*, consider the possibility that a member of your family could be a carrier and discuss this with your doctor.

4 Follow as many of the dietary recommendations in the Good Gut Upgrade (Chapter 2) as you possibly can. Improved diet is seen by many practitioners as a good way to deter *H. pylori*. In particular, give up cow's milk products and change to sheep's or goat's milk yoghurts and cheeses. Also, avoid wheat-bran breakfast cereals, sweet sugary foods and anything high in processed fat.

5 During treatment, consider other helpful natural alternatives to use alongside prescribed medication:

- Invest in a jar of high-factor Comvita Manuka Honey (UMF 20+ or 25+) and take it every day, either by the teaspoonful or on food. This product is expensive but proven to be antibacterial and I would very strongly recommend it for this condition.

- Use fresh garlic in your cooking and also consider taking a top-notch garlic supplement. Garlic has well-established antibacterial qualities.

- Mastic gum, available in capsule form, is a very potent inhibitor of *Helicobacter* (see Resources).

- Flavonoid supplements have been shown to have anti-*Helicobacter* properties.

6 Add herbs and spices, such as parsley, chilli and turmeric, to your meals. Studies show that they help to reduce *H. pylori* bacteria.

7 Don't forget that smoking and alcohol can both disturb the balance of acid. If you're suffering with, or being treated for, ulcers, it really is better to steer clear of cigarette smoke and watch the alcohol intake. Stick to no more than one unit of good wine per day and quit beer and spirits totally.

8 Make personal hygiene a priority and don't share cups, glasses or cutlery without washing them thoroughly in between.

9 Deal with stress. Helicobacter infection may be at the root of the problem but stress can still aggravate ulcers.

10 Chew your food really thoroughly and sit down to meals. Gulping food, eating on the run or bending, stretching and lifting too soon after eating can produce exactly the same symptoms as over-acidity. There is no point in taking acid-suppressing medication unless it's absolutely essential, and in many cases the best remedy is in looking after the digestion a bit more carefully.

11 Follow a course of probiotics as described in Chapter 7 on antibiotics. Don't forget that the recommended medical treatment for *Helicobacter pylori* infection will disturb the balance of good gut bacteria, which will then need to be supported and replaced.

Take care

Because the pain and discomfort of under-acidity and excess acidity are similar, the danger is that sufferers of under-acid stomachs can find themselves being treated routinely for excess acid, even if the opposite is true. It's also very common to find patients who are 'stuck' with prescriptions for long-term acid-suppressing medication even though the *H. pylori* may no longer be a problem or was never a problem in the first place. I regularly see patients who tell me that they've been told to take acid suppressors 'for life' when, in fact, doing so is not always necessary and, in some cases, is downright irresponsible. This is why it can be helpful to have tests to determine not only whether *H. pylori* is present but also to check the level of stomach acid that applies before treatment is commenced.

Be aware that anti-ulcer medicines can also mask *H. pylori* symptoms. In other words, you could be suffering from an overgrowth of this bacteria and not be aware of it. They are also known to affect the absorption of some minerals. If you are taking proton pump inhibitors or H2 receptor antagonists, make sure that you are seen regularly by your GP.

21.

Probiotics for Bladder and Vaginal Health

'The health benefits for which probiotics can be applied include conditions such as gastrointestinal infections, certain bowel disorders, allergy, and urogenital infections, which afflict a large portion of the world's population. The application of probiotics to prevent and treat these disorders should be more widely considered by the medical community. '

Joint FAO/WHO Expert Consultation, Codex Alimentarius Commission,
1–4 October 2001

Infections that set up home 'down there', whether they're in the bladder, urinary tract or vagina, can be a persistent nuisance. If you're reading this, chances are pretty high that you've had more than your fair share of burning discomfort, vaginal discharge or post-antibiotic thrush, not to mention the physical and emotional distress that goes with them.

Don't panic

If you're a sufferer of urine infections, thrush or bacterial vaginosis, you're not alone. It's estimated that, at any one time, more than three-quarters of the female population could have an imbalance of vaginal flora and may not even know it. Staggering though it sounds, figures for 2008 suggest that around 30 million women in North America will get some kind of urogenital infection. Anything that disturbs that bacterial balance (think antibiotics and other medicines such as steroids, anti-ulcer drugs and spermicides, inadequate fluid intake, not-so-good health, horrible hormones and excessive stress) can make picking up a water or vaginal infection really easy.

In case you're not familiar with these miserable conditions, here's what to watch for:

Urinary tract infections

A urinary tract infection or UTI[JB] is the general term used to indicate an infection of the bladder, urethra (the 'peeing pipe'), kidneys or ureters (the tubes that carry urine from the kidneys to the bladder). Symptoms can include:

- Discoloured, cloudy or foul-smelling urine.
- A feeling of pressure or sharp pain in the groin or region of the pubic bone.
- Persistent sensation of needing to empty the bladder, accompanied by pain and burning during urination.
- Sweating and shivering.
- Disturbed sleep.
- General lethargy and tiredness.

> **Jargon buster**
>
> Although urine is a waste product, it isn't supposed to contain anything very much in the way of bacteria. But when pathogenic bugs find their way via the urethra to the bladder or kidneys, that's when you can find yourself with a urinary tract infection, or **UTI**. The most familiar type of UTI is cystitis. Something with similar symptoms but harder to treat (and very often not involving bacteria) is trigonitis, inflammation of the lower part of the bladder.
>
> UTIs can occur in anyone at any age but tend to be more likely in sexually active women, in diabetics, men with prostate problems, the elderly, people with poor genital hygiene and in those who don't drink enough fluids. They

> can also be a nuisance to those with nervous-system disorders, and anyone with restricted movement such as someone confined to a wheelchair or long-term bed rest.

Take special note if you're elderly

In elderly people who suffer UTIs, problems with balance and unsteadiness on the feet are common. This is worth knowing, because they are symptoms often missed or simply associated with ageing. Given that there has long been concern about the repeated or excessive use of antibiotics in older people, it's just as well to wait for test results before resorting to these drugs. If tests show that medical treatment is not necessary, but symptoms still persist, then it's a good idea to check fluid intake, which, in the elderly, is often found to be far too low.

Kidney health

Untreated bladder and urethra infections can progress to kidney infection, such as polynephritis, which is not only more difficult to eradicate but can also lead to kidney damage. Infection of the kidneys may also be the result of bacteria passing through the kidneys from the bloodstream or could be the result of kidney stones.

In kidney infection, there may be:

- Any or all of the symptoms for urinary tract infections above.
- Back pain just above the waistband, pain in the side or in the lower abdomen.
- Extreme tiredness.
- High fever.
- Nausea or vomiting.
- Night sweats.

Avoiding kidney stones

Kidney stones are formed from crystals – most usually made up of calcium and another substance, called oxalate – that build up in the urine. Small crystals may be passed unnoticed but, sometimes, they accumulate into one or more larger pieces, which can irritate the kidneys and cause infection, damage or blockage. To give you some idea of how immobilising this can be, the pain caused by a kidney stone, especially if it's on the move, has very often been described as being akin to that of childbirth.

Although larger stones will almost inevitably require some kind of surgical intervention, small ones may work their way out of the body without major incident. The best-case scenario is to take preventive action to stop them occurring in the first place. Avoid excessive intakes of foods that are high in oxalate, such as spinach, rhubarb and wheat-bran cereals, and drink more fluid, which dilutes the urine and reduces the risk of particles accumulating. But now, a new probiotic discovery may give us another weapon against stone formation (see the action plan on page 234).

Bacterial vaginosis

Also called BV, bacterial vaginosis is the most common cause of vaginal infection (called vaginitis) and is believed to affect around one-third of all women aged between 15 and 50. It's recently been suggested that a major trigger may turn out to be a little-known bug called *Atopobium vaginae*. BV is twice as common as the yeast overgrowth candidiasis with which it is often confused. However, candidiasis is not caused by bacteria, and nor is thrush (which is why antibiotics don't work against *Candida albicans* and why anti-fungals don't work against BV), although probiotics can be helpful for 'yeasty' conditions.

More often than not, you'll need a swab test to determine an accurate diagnosis of bacterial vaginosis. Although often considered a sexually transmitted disease (STD), BV can occur where there's disruption of beneficial bacteria and a disturbance of the acid balance (pH) of the vagina. Common BV symptoms include:

- Heavy vaginal discharge.
- Fishy smelling discharge.
- Intense itching.

- Swelling around the labia.
- Abdominal cramp.

Antibiotic overkill?

It used to be the case that most urinary tract infections could be dispatched relatively quickly and effectively with a course of antibiotics. Unfortunately, now that antibiotic resistance has become such a feature of our lives, standard treatment can sometimes be counter-productive, often requiring several courses of antibiotics instead of one, as well as increasing the risk of another side effect: thrush. And even then, they might not work. The results of a number of different researches suggest that the right type of probiotic therapy, alone or in combination with other remedies, could provide us with a truly worthwhile alternative to antibiotic treatment and a real breakthrough in the management of recurring urinary tract and vaginal infections.

What if you have a negative urine test?

Sometimes, you might go down with one or more of the symptoms in the lists above and yet find that your urine test came back negative (showing no bacteria present). If that happens, it could indicate:

- Interstitial cystitis.
- Trigonitis.
- Non-bacterial cystitis or urethritis.
- Unrecognised or unusual viruses or bacteria present, *Chlamydia trachomatis* or *Neisseria gonorrheae* infection.
- In men, urinary frequency or painful urination (known as dysuria) associated with prostate inflammation.

Is your anatomy to blame?

Most of the bacteria that inhabit the urogenital areas of the body come from the gastrointestinal tract. Given the close proximity of the exit tubes for excreta and urine (and in women, the adjacent vaginal opening), it shouldn't come as much of a surprise to find that urinary and vaginal infections have often been linked to bad bacteria that began their journey in the large intestine (the colon). It's known that faecal microbes are found in the vagina. This is perfectly normal. The difference is that, in healthy subjects, the *Lactobacilli* family have the upper hand, whereas in women suffering infections, bad bacteria are in the majority. But think about this: if pathogenic microbes can sneak so easily 'round the corner', then why not good bacteria – which, of course, also live in and pass through the colon?

There are several studies linking beneficial bacteria with the health of the urinary system and which show that a regular supply of friendly flora could be one of the best ways of lessening the likelihood not only of cystitis but also of bacterial vaginosis. Research seems to suggest that good gut bugs, especially certain strains of *Lactobacilli*, set up home in the vagina and act as a protective barrier against any unwanted pathogens who might decide to take a day out and travel in the wrong direction.

Topping up the good guys at the diet end of things is also a good idea. The daily intake of a fresh live yoghurt or yoghurt drink is known to be beneficial for the bladder and vagina.

Action plan for urinary or vaginal problems

Act quickly and follow the suggestions below:

1 See your doctor or practice nurse if you suspect either a urinary or vaginal problem. Don't ignore the symptoms. Untreated urine infections can lead to kidney damage, and untreated BV could increase the risk of more serious conditions such as pelvic inflammatory disease. But don't accept antibiotics without vaginal swabs and/or urine tests being taken, otherwise you could end up with the wrong diagnosis and the wrong medication. There are several symptoms that can mimic infection but that don't require antibiotics. Vaginal discharge might, indeed, mean BV, which is an infection, but it could also suggest thrush, which isn't. Likewise, symptoms identical to those of a water infection might, as suggested above, be non-bacterial trigonitis, interstitial cystitis or an STD. A negative result may also indicate a viral condition or the presence of some kind of rarely seen bacteria. So it's important to be sure that you don't make matters worse by taking wrong or unnecessary prescription or over-the-counter drugs.

2 The medical literature tells us that recurrence of bacterial vaginosis is common in patients who have been prescribed the antibacterial drug metronidazole. If this sounds like you, then tell your doctor. If you seem to be getting repeated infections but don't know if you have ever taken this particular drug, ask the doctor or practice nurse to check your notes. Talk to your pharmacist. In addition to prescribed antibiotics, there are several products available over the counter that can help reduce symptoms. Some are designed to lower the pH of the vagina (which makes life uncomfortable for bad bacteria); others are naturally antibacterial and/or anti-fungal. There are also plenty of cranberry-based powders and drinks (avoid any that contain sugar), vaginal applicators containing healthy flora, helpful nutritional sugars and, of course, probiotic supplements.

3 Include live yoghurts or yoghurt drinks in your diet every day. And add plenty of other fermented and prebiotic foods. There is really good evidence available that fermented foods are valuable in the prevention and treatment of infections and yeast overgrowth.

4 If you're plagued on a regular basis with UTIs or vaginal thrush, invest in a top-quality probiotic and take it at least until symptoms are eradicated and then, as a maintenance dose, for a month every couple of months. Although there have been a few studies showing no benefit to using probiotic bacteria in the treatment of UTIs, the majority are extremely positive. I can certainly confirm excellent results in clinical practice with patients who had previously suffered from repeat infections. Other research does seem to substantiate that when good gut bugs are in short supply, the risk of urinary tract infections is higher.

> **Case history**
>
> It's not only scientific research that has confirmed the positive benefits of friendly flora like *Lactobacilli* in helping to prevent or treat urinary infections and yeast overgrowth. There's plenty of anecdotal evidence that slapping live yoghurt onto your bits gets good bugs into those difficult-to-reach places.
>
> This little case history might make you smile, told to me by the patient concerned. Her doctor advised her to get as much *Lactobacillus acidophilus* into her vagina as possible to help ease the vaginal thrush she'd contracted after antibiotics for a urinary infection. But she had difficulty, 'because the yoghurt kept spilling everywhere', until her husband came up with the idea of pouring the yoghurt into the vagina using a plastic funnel. 'It definitely did the trick,' she explained, 'and a week of applications cured the thrush, although we couldn't stop laughing about how someone might react if they had walked in on us!'

5 In addition to any other treatment you may be using to treat vaginal infections, you might also try mixing a couple of tablespoons of live yoghurt (plain, no sugar or additives) with the contents of a probiotic capsule or single serving of probiotic powder (ideally one that includes *Lactobacillus acidophilus*), sloshing the whole lot into a bidet or bowl of tepid water and using it as a daily douche. But don't get confused that vaginal and urine infections can be cured by excessive cleanliness. Although good hygiene is a given, over-douching can make matters worse by washing out any good bacteria. Everyone carries yeast organisms, which live naturally within us, so it isn't realistic to try to eradicate them. The key to comfort is control.

6 Consider a course of probiotics, too, if you're pregnant or breastfeeding. Studies show that breastfeeding can reduce the risk of UTIs in babies and may confer greater protection in later life against this condition. In addition, certain *Lactobacillus* strains, such as *Lactobacilli rhamnosus* and *Lactobacilli reuteri* have been shown to be helpful to pregnant women suffering from bacterial vaginosis and could even be more effective than antibiotics. According to Gregor Reid, Professor of Microbiology and Immunology at The University of Western Ontario, a course of supplements could have the desired effect in three to five days and, encouragingly, that suppositories (if and when available) could work even more quickly.

7 It's been discovered that people prone to calcium oxalate kidney stones tend to have lower levels of a particularly helpful bacteria called *Oxalobacter formigenes*, which is involved in making an enzyme that breaks down the oxalates. Replacing *O. formigenes* isn't an option because it's not available as a supplement. However, other familiar and easily obtained probiotics, *Bifidobacterium infantis*, *Bifidobacterium lactis* and *Lactobacillus acidophilus*, could ride to the rescue because they, too, are able to manufacture the missing enzyme.

8 Read Chapter 11 on allergies. Adverse reactions to certain foods can cause urinary-tract inflammation by irritating the bladder wall.

9 Drink more water. A low intake of fluid definitely increases the risk of infection because it concentrates the urine. Increasing your intake throughout the day is obvious common sense but drinking an additional glass of water first thing in the morning before breakfast may also be especially helpful.

10 Girls: don't wear thongs; they're notorious for triggering urogenital problems because of the irritation caused by fabric chafing. For the same reason, it's best to get used to life without tight jeans. And avoid underwear made from non-breathable fibres.

11 Go for bleach-free sanitary protection such as the 100 per cent organic cotton range from Natracare. They make pads, towels, tampons and wet wipes, all biodegradable and free from chlorine, sodium laurel sulphate, parabens and perfumes, which are all potential allergens.

12 Pay sensible attention to genital hygiene:

- Keep your bits clean. This applies particularly after a bowel movement, and before and after intercourse.

- Don't hang on and put it off when you need to urinate. When you're done, always wipe from front to back.

- Empty your bladder after sex. Even if all you really want to do is to roll over and go to sleep, making the effort to go to the bathroom means that you help flush accumulated bacteria away rather than leaving it there to multiply. Washing thoroughly around the opening to the vagina and urethra has been shown to reduce the risk of infection occurring, but don't get carried away with excess douching or the use of highly antiseptic vaginal products.

Other remedies worth considering:

1 Acupuncture is said to be helpful in the treatment of recurrent urinary infections. There are a handful of studies showing good results and, in addition, patient feedback is positive. It's certainly worth a go, especially if you're at the end of your tether and nothing else is working.

2 There seems little doubt that cranberry is beneficial in reducing attacks of cystitis for some people and can be especially useful for those who suffer regular episodes of urinary infection. You may be one who swears by cranberry juice, and if it works for you then that's great. Unfortunately, most cartons or bottles of cranberry have a high sugar content, which can aggravate thrush, so if that bothers you then it may be better to source sugar-free concentrated cranberry in capsules or liquid. It can be even more effective if taken in conjunction with a probiotic. I have also found that decent daily doses of vitamin C complex (those that come with flavonoids, not the plain ascorbic acid tablets that you dissolve in water) are as good, if not better, than cranberry. I usually recommend 2g three times daily during an attack and 1g daily as a maintenance dose. I've included cranberry-based supplements and vitamin C supplements in Resources.

Unfortunately, cranberry is not helpful for everyone and, in fact, in a few cases that I've seen, it has actually made matters worse. If it doesn't suit you, the following paragraphs may be of special interest.

3 Herbal remedies can provide valuable support. I would always consider Dr Vogel's Echinaforce as a number-one helper. Use the tincture rather than the tablets. I find it works more quickly, and because it's a liquid that you need to take with water, it helps you to increase that all-important fluid intake. Also useful is the herb uva-ursi, which has antiseptic and anti-inflammatory properties. If you're a person who is plagued by repeated attacks of cystitis, then these two plant remedies are worth using regularly as prevention.

4 The whey drink Molkosan has a natural antibiotic action and is prebiotic, so it encourages repopulation of healthy bacteria in the urinary tract. It's also soothing for that sharp pain associated with urinary infection and is an excellent therapy for dealing with thrush.

Glyconutrients

Another way of knocking urinary tract infections on the head is by using something called glyconutrients, also called nutritional sugars. If you suffer repeatedly from cystitis, then this is a very worthwhile treatment, especially if you've reached the stage where you think nothing is ever going to work or you're battling with the misery of repeated infections that haven't responded to antibiotics.

Although we usually think of sugar, such as sucrose, as being damaging to the body (ordinary table sugar is sucrose), some types are actually beneficial. When it comes to treating intractable urinary infections, I have seen excellent results for d-mannose.

The 'd' in d-mannose stands for 'dextra' (think dextrose), which indicates that it's a sugar. The way that bad bacteria actually set up an infection is first to get a grip onto the bladder wall. When we take d-mannose as a supplement, the excess mannose washes through the bladder and the bad guys don't like it. Suddenly unable to hang on any longer, undesirable bacteria, such as pathogenic *E. coli*, simply get flushed out of the body when we urinate.

D-mannose doesn't kill bacteria – it just prevents them from latching on to you. Because it also has anti-inflammatory properties, it's extremely valuable in treating non-bacterial cystitis, painful bladder syndrome, interstitial cystitis and trigonitis.

D-mannose is a relatively unknown but an extremely beneficial and safe treatment that works well in arresting persistent cases of urinary infection and inflammation. However, for some people with very sensitive bladders prone to repeated attack, it does need to be taken very regularly, which can get expensive. My experience as a practitioner has been that, when used alongside a single two-month course of high-dose (20 billion) probiotics, the length of treatment tends to be shorter and doesn't need to be repeated so often, sometimes not at all. I have to stress that this is only my personal experience of its usefulness in actual practice with a mere handful of patients and I have no scientific studies to confirm my findings. However, it may be something for you to consider.

There's more information in Resources.

22.

Good Gut Bugs for Mums and Babies

Although there is undeniable evidence of the value of probiotics in repopulating the intestines that support our health, of course the absolute best time to ensure the healthiest possible gut conditions is at the beginning of life, not partway through it.

At the very moment before we are born, our digestive systems are sterile. Not a bug in sight. Here's where we have our golden opportunity to start as we mean to go on.

Being born is a thoroughly messy experience, but I wonder though how many people consider the fact that the muckier the mess, the healthier the baby is likely to be? Or that the route it takes to reach the outside world could make the difference between a strong immune system or one that's destined to struggle?

There seems to be little doubt but that the conditions surrounding a baby's birth and its immediate aftercare are enough to determine which types of bacteria they're exposed to in the early days of life and, in turn, are one of the major influences in the long-term make-up of their intestinal microflora.

Natural birth

Arrive via the normal, natural route, and a baby will pick up bacteria from the mother's vagina and from her involuntary faecal waste. This may sound unclean but, in fact, it's exactly what the baby needs, especially as the beneficial bugs are likely to include strains such as *Bifidobacteria* and *Lactobacillus*. In its first few hours and days, the little one will also gather bacteria which we normally think of as not so nice, such as certain *Streptococcus, Escherichia coli* (*E. coli*) and *Staphylococcus aureus*, picked up from the mother's skin, from feeding, handling by parents and others, kisses and cuddles from doting relatives and in general from the surrounding environment. This is all entirely normal and should give the baby the proper balance of microflora with which to begin life outside the mother's sterile womb.

Beneficial bugs not included

A baby that's lifted out of the uterus by Caesarean section will also collect some of its mother's microbes but, unfortunately, the majority of bacteria are far more likely to be of the hospital variety, unable to provide the newborn with the ideal immune-system support. Whereas the breast-fed baby becomes well populated with *Bifidobacteria*, the intestinal flora of formula-fed infants is far more wide ranging and will also include higher numbers of *Streptococci*, *Enterococci* and *Clostridia*. Similarly, in premature and low-birthweight babies, the gut flora tends to be dominated by strains of *Enterococci, E. coli, Staphylococci* and *Klebsiella*. It's just this kind of bacterial soup that has been found in the intestines of infants and young children who go on to develop allergies. One reason for this could be that, because our friendly flora have such an important role to play in preparing or training our immune systems to fight invaders, a lack of good gut bugs leaves it untrained and unprimed, and therefore probably more inclined to overreact when an allergen comes along. Work is ongoing to find out if the differences in gut flora might also be the result of allergies rather than a cause.

On the negative side, exposure of babies and youngsters to antibiotics is known to upset the good gut flora, and research tells us that this not only increases the risk of conditions such as allergies, asthma and eczema but may also make susceptibility to other diseases more likely; for example, one study showed a link between imbalances of *Bacteroides* bacteria and ankylosing spondylitis, a painful and debilitating arthritic condition that affects the spine.

Breast really is best

According to the World Health Organization Regional Office for Europe, less than 35 per cent of all infants worldwide are exclusively breast-fed 'for even the first 4 months of life'. This means that around two-thirds of all newborns may be at a distinct disadvantage when it comes to programming their immunity for future good health. In a healthy newborn, *Bifidobacteria* will initially make up the majority of gut flora.

These beneficial bugs are further enhanced by proteins and other nutrients found in the mother's milk. Early on in life the natural sugars in mother's milk get converted into lactic acid, which is why, remember, they're called lactic acid bacteria. All this helps to prime the immune system so that it provides protection against infection while the baby is developing his or her own natural immunity. This is a situation that 'embeds' itself specifically during infancy, giving the body the ability to recognise and fight harmful bacteria and yet leave the beneficial bacteria untouched. Time seems to be of the essence here, since research suggests there may be only a relatively short window of opportunity during the first few weeks in which to ensure the best possible colonisation of the baby's intestines.

?

Did you know?
The World Health Organization and United Nations both recommend exclusive breastfeeding for the first six months, plus breastfeeding support during weaning for up to two years or beyond. And they give this useful advice to health professionals:

- Help mothers initiate breastfeeding within half an hour of birth.
- Show mothers how to breastfeed, and how to maintain lactation, even if they should be separated from their infants.
- Give newborn infants no food and drink other than breast milk, unless medically indicated.
- Practise rooming-in: allow mothers and infants to remain together 24 hours a day.

- Encourage breastfeeding on demand.
- Give no artificial teats or pacifiers (also called dummies or soothers) to breastfeeding infants.
- Foster the establishment of breastfeeding support groups and refer mothers to them on discharge from the hospital or clinic.

Caesarean section

Although there's no complete substitute for breast milk, the addition of probiotics to formula feeds may be especially good news for babies born by Caesarean section or who don't have the benefit of breastfeeding.

When you add surgical birth to a complete absence of breast-feeding and then top that off with time spent in a baby-care unit, perhaps followed by repeated use of antibiotics, then any chance that healthy gut flora might have had of doing a good job could have been completely wiped out.

Sometimes, of course, a C-section is unavoidable and may be the end result of a complicated pregnancy and/or premature birth. Where babies have to be separated from their mothers and cared for in neonatal units, it can be days or weeks before they can be breastfed, or they may never benefit from breastfeeding at all. This means that the gut is more at risk from being colonised by unwelcome bacteria, which can lead not only to the increased risk of asthma and allergies but more immediately to a life-threatening condition known as necrotising enterocolitis. Already, a number of studies using probiotics for premature babies have shown a decrease in the number of cases of this life-threatening condition and improvements in survival rates.

By the way, something that's not always emphasised is that these important beneficial microbes don't thrive so well on cow's milk formula, leaving the child more at risk from infections and the aforementioned allergies.

An ideal world

Ideally, we would all arrive by natural childbirth and be breastfed exclusively for at least six months. I know I will always be grateful to my mum who, although she worked full time, breastfed me for two years. She tells me it was because it was free! But the upshot is that her daughter has a healthy gut and a strong immunity. Although there's clearly no substitute for mother's milk and the bacterial benefits that it provides, at least probiotic foods and supplements are now widely available for both adults and little ones. Although some trials found probiotics to make little or no difference, many other studies show that the potential benefits to mums and babies of taking probiotics is impressive:

- Taking probiotic foods such as yoghurts, fermented milks and aged cheeses can help to improve the transit time of food through the gut, easing constipation and reducing gas.

- Adding *Bifidobacteria* and *Lactobacillus* to premature infant feeding can reduce the risk of necrotising enterocolitis.

- Allergic mums who take probiotics during pregnancy and continue to use them through breastfeeding may lessen the risk of that allergy profile being passed to the breastfed baby.

- Probiotics given to pregnant mums for two to four weeks before delivery and then also to the newborn babies (who were followed by the study until age four) showed a 50 per cent drop in recurring atopic eczema.

- Probiotic supplements taken during pregnancy can also help to prevent the severe constipation so commonly associated with pregnancy and, as a result, reduce the risk of piles (haemorrhoids).

- Probiotics may help towards better growth development in children.

- Pregnant mothers suffering the discomfort of bacterial vaginosis could also benefit from taking supplements of friendly flora (see page 233).

- In babies and young children given antibiotics for respiratory infections, probiotics were able to reduce the incidence of antibiotic-related diarrhoea.

- Babies who suffer from colic generally have lower levels of good gut bugs. In bottle-fed babies, supplementing formula with probiotics can help ease colic.

- Breastfeeding can reduce the risk of urinary tract infections in infants.

- Breastfeeding and probiotic supplements can both be useful in the treatment of acute rotavirus (see page 209).

- Giving probiotic supplements to toddlers may help reduce the risk of picking up repeated infections in child-care centres and pre-school nursery.

> **!**
>
> ### Very important point
> When choosing probiotics for babies and young children, always ask advice either from a qualified practitioner who is familiar with their use or get data direct from the manufacturer. This is important, because the strains of bacteria suitable for newborns and toddlers are different from those recommended for adults. *Bifidobacterium infantis* is one that is available for newborns. For toddlers and growing children up to ten years old, combination products that include *Lactobacillus acidophilus* and *Bifidobacterium bifidum* have produced good results especially where there was poor immunity to infection, skin problems or allergies. (Recommended suppliers appear in Resources.)

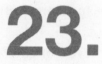

Can Probiotics Help Other Gut Disorders?

'Probiotics provide an extra layer of strength. [They behave like] soldiers in your intestinal tract to combat pathogens ...'

Dr Mary Ellen Sanders, expert in probiotic microbiology

This section may be helpful if you suffer from:

- Leaky gut syndrome
- Candidiasis
- Crohn's disease
- Ulcerative colitis

Leaky gut syndrome

The condition, leaky gut syndrome, is defined as 'an increase in permeability of the lining of the intestines to large food molecules, antigens (foreign invaders) and toxins, leading to inflammation, cell destruction and mucosal damage'. It's nearly always associated with poor digestion, where foods are not broken down properly and the lining of the intestines becomes irritated and inflamed, affecting the permeability[JB] of the gut wall. In other words, it gets full of holes that allow undigested food, bacteria and toxins to leak into the bloodstream. Not surprisingly, this causes the immune system to react to what it thinks are alien invaders, triggering a whole load of other extremely unpleasant symptoms.

Although not readily acknowledged by conventional medicine, leaky gut syndrome is considered by many naturopaths and nutrition-oriented doctors as a major cause of disease and has been implicated in a long list of health problems, such as candidiasis, chronic fatigue, food allergies, gluten sensitivity, headaches, migraine, intestinal parasites, irritable bowel syndrome, chronic sinusitis, and even certain types of depression.

Jargon buster

The best way to describe **permeability** is to picture the gut wall as a protective barrier between the intestines and the bloodstream, full of tiny perforations or pores, just like a sieve or a strainer, only much smaller. Only substances that have the right 'keys' – such as nutrients – are allowed to pass from one side to the other. But if the gut is irritated or inflamed, the holes can be damaged or enlarged and the membrane becomes more 'holey', allowing undigested food, bacteria and other unwanted particles, to get into the blood system, increasing the risk of allergic reactions and a condition known as leaky gut syndrome.

Too many bad bacteria?

No one yet knows the actual cause except that a 'holey' gut might be the result of a defect caused by an overgrowth of bacteria. On the gut wall itself, there are only so many spaces available for bacteria to snuggle down. Put simply, if good gut bugs are in short supply or non-existent in the gut, pathogenic bacteria will multiply and take up all the available room. When this happens, the gut wall reacts by becoming inflamed. Results from animal studies seem to suggest that supplementing probiotics and restoring the balance of good gut bugs could help to heal the gut wall by preventing pathogens sticking to the surface and reducing intestinal inflammation (see page 260). The successful results of using probiotics in practice would appear to confirm these findings, so let's hope for more research.

Candidiasis and related yeasty beasties

In Chapter 21, we talked about how probiotics can help thrush. They can be valuable in other yeast-related conditions, too, including fungal infections of the groin (jock itch), of the feet (sometimes known as athlete's foot), fungal nails and the serious gut disorder known as candidiasis. Even though research is still limited, the empirical evidence showing probiotics to be helpful as part of the treatment for this widespread condition is overwhelming.

Anyone who suffers, or has suffered, with chronic candidiasis will already know that it's not a syndrome that is recognised by a majority of the medical profession. They acknowledge the yeast *Candida albicans* and that yeast overgrowth occurs in immune-compromised patients, such as those with cancer or AIDS. They also obviously agree upon the existence of vaginal and oral thrush and fungal infections of the skin. But because there is no direct scientific proof that chronic candidiasis exists as an illness in its own right, many sufferers find themselves either out in the cold with no medical support or otherwise branded with a psychosomatic disorder. Although there is scientific research being carried out into the involvement of *Candida albicans* in other diseases, there are no direct studies being done, nor are there, at the moment, any trials looking at probiotics in relation to candidiasis. However, despite all this, practitioners who specialise in its treatment continue to see a steady stream of candidiasis sufferers. If it was all psychosomatic, one has to ask why the tried-and-tested treatments for this condition are so effective.

About candida

Just in case you're not sure, *Candida albicans* is the Latin name of the yeast fungus itself. Candidiasis is the term used to describe the chronic condition that invades and affects the whole body. It's also sometimes called candida related complex, or CRC, although the word 'candida' is often used on its own as an abbreviation for both the yeast and for the condition it causes.

Everybody has candida yeast in their system; under normal circumstances it's a benign inhabitant of the intestines, just like

246

many of the bacteria that we've been talking about throughout *Good Gut Bugs*, which, if left alone to get on with their normal tasks, behave themselves and do no harm. Again, just like those bacteria, in certain situations where the status quo is disrupted, this simple yeast changes from Dr Jekyll into Mr Hyde, turning on the healthy membranes between the intestines and the bloodstream, damaging the gut wall and allowing toxins to seep into the general circulation. By the way, a leaky gut is commonplace in CRC.

Candidiasis can affect anyone at any age, although it's believed to be around eight times more likely to occur in women than in men simply because it's aggravated by increased use of antibiotics for conditions such as cystitis, by the birth control pill and hormone replacement therapy. There are many other triggers, too, and the list is long and depressing. Most sufferers can point to:

- Repeated or long-term use of antibiotics; that is, for acne or urinary infections.
- Food sensitivities/allergies.
- Headaches or migraine.
- Lethargy or chronic fatigue.
- A range of gastrointestinal symptoms that may include bloating, flatulence, constipation, diarrhoea, and the general feeling of 'unwellness' after eating.
- Impaired memory or poor recall, associated with feelings of being 'spaced out' and suffering 'brain fog'.
- Depression (hardly surprising).
- Absence of any other medical diagnosis.
- Improvements following the removal from the diet of certain foods, the use of anti-fungal treatments and the introduction of probiotics.

The role of probiotics

We know that probiotics have long been acknowledged by sufferers and their practitioners as an essential part of treatment. If they work so well for yeast overgrowth in other areas of the body then why not for the gut? In fact, any time that the body is invaded by an overgrowth of yeast, it's a fair bet that not only is the immune system likely to be under strain but that the levels of good gut bugs will have been compromised in some way.

Help for candidiasis

My first advice to anyone who thinks they might be suffering with chronic candidiasis would always be to find a qualified and empathetic practitioner who understands and specialises in treating the condition. In the meantime:

1 Remove all wheat products, especially bread and anything containing yeast, sugar, sugary foods, cow's milk and artificial food additives from your existing diet.

2 Steer well clear of alcohol. Not only does it aggravate the condition but it also puts additional strain on your liver, which is already having to deal with the 'internal' alcohol being fuelled by the yeast itself.

3 Reduce chemical exposure by upgrading as much as possible to natural household cleaning fluids and natural skincare products.

4 Follow the advice on how to reduce the need for antibiotics (page 117) and the information concerning antibiotic resistance (page 114).

5 Focus on fresh vegetables, salads, oily fish and organic poultry.

6 Use garlic in your cooking.

7 Include plenty of fresh, plain live yoghurt, kefir, Molkosan, buttermilk and other prebiotic foods in the diet. Together with probiotics, these foods help to make the gut more acidic, which yeasts really don't like.

8 Take supplements that have natural anti-fungal and/or anti-parasitic properties, such as those made from grapefruit seed extract, caprylic acid, oregano, barberry bark, wormwood, clove and black walnut.

9 Invest in the best-quality probiotic you can afford.

> **!**
>
> **Very important point**
> The advice above may also be helpful for anyone troubled by persistent fungal infections of the skin or by repeated episodes of thrush.

Details of support for candida sufferers can be found at the end of the Resources section on page 288.

Inflammatory bowel disease

IBD – inflammatory bowel disease – is a general heading that includes Crohn's disease and ulcerative colitis (U/C), both serious intestinal conditions associated with diarrhoea, pain, poor absorption of nutrients and subsequent malnutrition, periods of hospitalisation and, in advanced cases, operations to remove parts of the colon. Generally, Crohn's disease affects the small intestine, although it can spread to the large intestine, whereas ulcerative colitis is restricted only to the large intestine. Both are characterised by flare-ups and periods of remission.

Interestingly, IBD is far more common in countries that have a high standard of living and where children are subjected to good hygiene in their early years. It is also linked to lack of breastfeeding and diets that are heavy on animal fats and sugar but light on fruits, vegetables and whole grains. Regular use of antibiotics in early life may be an added risk factor. The irony here is that because inflamed tissue often becomes infected, patients suffering IBD, especially those with Crohn's disease, frequently find themselves having to take yet more antibiotics and creating the inevitable vicious circle. Medical treatments also include antibody and immune-system suppressing drugs, although these are not ideal because of their toxicity.

What causes IBD?

Although the actual causes are not known, there may be a genetic component, since IBD can run in families. And although an infectious aspect has not been confirmed in humans, one animal study found that ulcerative colitis could be passed not only from mother to offspring but also between adult animals. Around one in five of patients suffering ulcerative colitis have a close relative with the disease or who suffers with Crohn's disease.

It may also be that there's some kind of intolerance to normal microflora in the gut, which then causes the inflammation associated with both conditions. Even if this turns out to be the case, no one yet knows whether we're talking about one troublesome bacterium or a whole community of different ones, or whether, perhaps, inflammation is some kind of precursor, which then upsets the bacteria. It is certainly true that the gut lining of IBD patients is more permeable, as it is in leaky gut syndrome, although, again, it's not clear whether the permeability causes the inflammation or the inflammation causes the permeability; or whether it's the immune system upsetting the bacteria, or vice versa.

Since both Crohn's and U/C could be disorders of the immune system linked to inflammation, and since beneficial bacteria have anti-inflammatory properties, it makes sense that administration of probiotics might prevent inflammation. The results of a number of clinical trials have demonstrated that certain strains of probiotics may be able to lengthen the periods of remission, although not all conclusions have been positive; for example, there are several studies in which probiotics just didn't make any difference. However, they have been used successfully in patients who've had part or all of the colon removed as a result of ulcerative colitis and also in a complication of IBD called pouchitis, an inflammation of a section of the remaining intestine. Other results show that probiotic supplementation may be just as effective as low-dose aspirin-based anti-inflammatory drugs.

New findings on ulcerative colitis

In the particular case of ulcerative colitis, one now famous study has found a deficiency of a particular peacekeeping cell – a type of regulating protein called T-bet – in the immune system, which leaves the way open for 'bad' bacteria to damage the gut wall and cause inflammation. T-bet proteins are involved in policing the borders (in this case the one between your gut and your bloodstream), capturing the 'identities' of foreign microbes. They check them at 'passport control' and then, if they think there might be a problem, they call up other immune defences. When T-bet levels are normal, the frontier holds firm and pathogenic bacteria give up trying to get across. Because there's no invasion, there's no inflammation either. But where the T-bet officers are missing, massive inflammation is triggered and normal cells die off. In ulcerative colitis, this damage to the gut wall appeared in 100 per cent of the animals involved in the study. This doesn't necessarily mean, of course, that the same results would apply in humans.

Further study is ongoing, but these early results do tend to confirm that there is some kind of variation in the DNA of people suffering ulcerative colitis. Although researchers have discovered that certain types of antibody drugs actually cured and prevented ulcerative colitis in their T-bet-deficient mice, the toxic side effects mean that their use is not ideal in humans. So now scientists are looking into other possible treatments, which include trying to directly manipulate the immune system by increasing T-bet levels or other immune-suppressing cells or by supplementing probiotics with the purpose of keeping harmful bacteria in check. This particular study hasn't identified any specific rabble-rousing bacteria, although it did rule out *E. Coli*, *H. pylori* and *Salmonella*. If nothing else, it confirms the complicated and vital relationship between the bacterial population of the intestines and the immune system that polices it. The laboratory concerned is now working to discover the likely troublemaker(s), which, it's already been suggested, could be one of the body's normally well-behaved natural inhabitants gone bad.

Treatments for IBD

Other research has shown that SCFAs (short chain fatty acids) can help to prevent IBD. SCFAs are produced by the process of fermentation in the colon, which relies not only on prebiotics being supplied in the diet but also on a healthy balance of beneficial bacteria. In particular, one type called butyrate, produced by fibre known as resistant starch (see Chapter 6), could be especially helpful because of its anti-inflammatory properties.

My own experience in treating patients with IBD has been very encouraging, but I'm not using probiotics in isolation, which is what tends to happen in scientific studies. Improved diet, concentrating on the removal of what I would call 'aggressive' dietary fibre and the introduction of more gentle prebiotic fibres, the addition of immune-boosting nutrients, Echinaforce tincture and probiotics have produced excellent results in what could only be described as extreme cases.

Help for IBD

Although there is not the space here to cover the subject of IBD in detail, I've included the main points of treatment below. I must stress, however, that these recommendations are based purely on personal experience in a clinical setting:

1 **Remove all wheat, wheat-bran cereals and cow's milk** from the diet. Avoid as far as possible any foods containing added sugar, artificial colourings, flavourings and sweeteners. Likewise, high-fat foods, and processed, packaged ready meals. Avoid completely all pork products including bacon, sausage and ham. Keep other red meat to a minimum.

2 **Avoid beer and spirits**. Some patients find that they can tolerate and enjoy an occasional glass of red wine or a vodka and soda, but if alcohol aggravates the condition, then it is obviously best avoided.

3 **Increase the intake of fruit and vegetables**, especially by making fresh juices and home-made soups. Fresh fruits and vegetables should make up at least one-third of the daily food intake. Red and purple fruits may be particularly helpful.

4 **Include fresh fish, plain live yoghurt, organic poultry and organic soya**. I stress the word 'organic' because non-organic produce may contain antibiotic and other chemical residues. Oily

fish, rich in omega-3, may be of special value; some research shows that patients who increased their intake of oily fish were able to reduce their anti-inflammatory medication. Sheep and goat's milk yoghurt and cheeses are also good protein sources that are generally better tolerated than cow's milk products.

5 Avoid sunflower oil, corn oil and processed margarine products. Use extra virgin olive oil for cooking and for salads.

6 Take Echinaforce tincture at 20 drops daily, increasing to twice daily if there is any infection present.

7 Take a basic multivitamin–mineral, preferably in liquid form (see Resources), with food.

8 Ensure a high fluid intake based on noncarbonated water, fresh juices, teas and broths.

9 Supplement broad-spectrum amino acid capsules to be taken before each meal. I would consider this an extremely important part of treatment. Currently, broad-spectrum amino acids are available from Biocare (see Resources). Amino acids are the building blocks of protein. For some reason, which is not yet clear, using these specialist supplements does seem to help some sufferers of IBD to improve their protein digestion.

10 Take a daily serving of fermented milk or a yoghurt product. The results of one small study suggested that strains of *Bifidobacterium breve* and *Bifidobacterium bifidum* with *Lactobacillus acidophilus* could be of value in encouraging remission in ulcerative colitis.

11 Introduce a daily probiotics supplement of *Lactobacillus acidophilus* and *Bifidobacterium* to be taken with milled flax (in this particular case, avoid flax*seed*) as per the instructions on page 99.

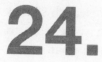

Inflammation, Immunity and Probiotics

We know from research done so far that where the immune system isn't functioning properly, the body's resistance to invasion by bad bacteria is seriously reduced. There's also evidence that maintaining good levels of friendly flora gives support to the immune system. But there's another angle here that may provide further clues as to the reasons behind certain illnesses. Have you ever noticed that an awful lot of diseases are associated with some kind of swelling, puffiness, hypersensitivity, pressure, or inflamed tissues? Fluid retention and arthritis are two that spring immediately to mind. But would it surprise you to know that inflammation is also an important factor in the health of the human body?

Most inflammatory responses are under the direct control of the immune system, and it's the immune system that stands between you and whether or not you get sick. That's why researchers are especially interested in any connection there may be between poor levels of good gut bugs and how this might affect the way the body deals with inflammation.

Encouragingly, results from this work show that probiotic foods and supplements could have the power to regulate or adjust the way we react to swelling, which is why I thought it might be helpful to give you a quick description of how your immune system functions.

Your immune system

We're talking here about one of the most complicated and complex body processes in the body. But to explain it to you in detail would take ages, and it isn't necessary for the purposes of this exercise. For now, let me give you a very brief description of where probiotics fit into the picture.

Security against invasion

Your immune system is your body's security against invasion by disease. Every time you put food or drink into your mouth, or you touch another human being or just simply breathe, you're exposed to bacteria. The reason you don't usually get sick and keel over is because your immune system shields and protects you. Most of it is controlled by a police force of dozens of different white blood cells that spend their lives operating undercover inside your body. They're everywhere, patrolling the roads and alleyways of your lymph system[JB] and your bloodstream, keeping an eye out for unwanted microbes: the bad guys.

> **Jargon buster**
>
> The **lymph system** is the network of vessels that weaves in and around the blood vessels, carrying lymph fluid to the circulation – a bit like country lanes that criss-cross main roads and go under and over motorways.
>
> **Lymph fluid** is a clear or slightly yellow liquid substance that is charged with white blood cells.
>
> **Lymph nodes** are like junctions in the lymph system where white blood cells congregate, waiting to attack invaders. These are the 'swollen glands' in the sides of your throat and under your arms that you can sometimes feel if you have an infection.

These 'officers' are especially busy in the area of the digestive system. Something in the order of 70–75 per cent of our immune system is based in the intestines. It's easy to see why: it's a good vantage point. This is where they have the best view of anything travelling down through the gastrointestinal tract (explained on page 57). The food that we eat, the saliva we swallow, all the gunge that rolls down the back of the nose or out of the sinus cavities and, of course, the air we take in, are all potential carriers of bacteria, viruses, parasites, yeasts and other unwanted pathogens, and are all, eventually, going to pass through the stomach and into the intestines.

Security alert!

When bacteria threaten to invade the body – say you picked up a cold virus from someone who sneezed over you – an alarm goes off that alerts the uniform branch to attend the incident. They're the interceptors, out on the streets constantly looking for trouble-makers. They turn up in an instant and make a speedy assessment of the situation. One of the first things they do is to check the 'most wanted' database in their computers to see if this criminal has been active in the vicinity in the past. If it has (in other words, you might have had a similar virus before), it's just a matter of calling in special forces who have all the information they need on this particular perpetrator, allowing them to deal quietly and efficiently with the matter – and you won't even have known there was a problem. The cold passed you by.

But if this is a new invader, they'll almost certainly call for back-up. First to arrive will be the fire brigade, who rush in with their hoses, which gush fluid into the area that has been attacked. Their quick-thinking action brings increased blood flow and other watery liquids to the site, carrying bacteria-killing cells and making the tissues tender and hot (hence the swelling). In the case of a cold, for example, this explains your painful sinuses, blocked nose and the problems you're having with swallowing. These areas are inflamed. The other things that often get swollen, of course, are the lymph glands, a discomfort caused by white blood cells that are queuing up in your lymph nodes, ready to attack.

If you cut your finger or foot on something sharp while you were in the garden, a similar thing happens. The skin swells up around the site of the injury. Then things really get busy. An army of experts is called in. Suspects are arrested or they get poisoned with chemical weapons (a kind of internal biological warfare) or they're eaten (nice). Unfortunately, sometimes, innocent bystanders are caught in the fray and get injured or killed. All this results in discarded blood cells, tissue debris and bacteria that form into the thick yellowish fluid we call pus.

Once the danger is passed, the police hand over to other specialist cells that are in charge of cooling the inflammation. They tell the cells in charge of the swelling to stand down; their job is done, the scene of crime is cleared, fever subsides, puffiness dissipates and everything is back to normal.

Very important point

A rise in body temperature is often assumed to be a bad thing, and we are usually advised to take paracetamol or a cold remedy to help reduce it. But the fever that comes with the illness is part of the immune system's response. Bacteria don't enjoy very cold temperatures, but they don't like hot conditions either. In fact, they thrive best at body temperature. The immune system knows this and so it pushes up your body temperature by a couple of degrees or so in order to make it much more difficult for the bad bacteria to multiply.

Take care

What's important to remember is that very high temperatures, especially in babies, children, teens, twenties and the elderly, are likely to be dangerous. If you're unsure, call the doctor without delay.

Acceleration and inflammation

One of the best analogies of how inflammation affects the body that I have ever heard is to liken it to the speed of a car. It works like this: when you press down on the accelerator, a cable sends a signal to the immune system, which revs up and triggers inflammation. Put a foot on the brake pedal and the immune system gets the message to cool it, to stop the inflammation. But sometimes there's a fault and it doesn't stop. It keeps right on going, just like stepping on the accelerator and 'flooring it' and then finding to your horror that your foot is stuck or you can't locate the brake. Like a car out of control, an immune system that's in permanent overdrive is also heading for disaster, which is why inflammatory diseases so often end up 'crashing' the body into serious ill-health or even total demise. In other words, normal inflammatory responses are essential to our recovery from illness or injury, but abnormal responses are like repeatedly wrecking the car.

As you might already have guessed, there's much more to all this than a cut or a cold. While the immune system is extremely clever at spotting invaders, sometimes it registers a normal cell or normal substance as a danger and instead of turning the inflammation switch to OFF, it ignores the instruction and carries on producing the chemicals that caused the reaction in the first place. This is what happens in the allergic reactions that we talk about on page 155. And it's this type of reaction that's implicated in serious auto-immune disorders such as rheumatoid arthritis, Crohn's disease, multiple sclerosis and type-1 (sometimes called junior-onset) diabetes. Researchers are also now beginning to wonder if a kind of lower level of chronic inflammation might explain other conditions such as fibromyalgia, obesity and syndromes such as chronic fatigue syndrome (ME) and irritable bowel (IBS).

Inflammation and cancer

The situation is slightly different, but nonetheless serious, in cancer, where cells have mutated (changed their appearance). Every day in every human being, there's the very strong likelihood that potentially dangerous cancerous cells are produced. Where the immune system is switched on and behaving normally, those cells will quickly be located and destroyed. But when the change in the cell structure is only very slight, the officers in charge of the tracking may have difficulty matching the photo-fit picture to the real villain. As a result, the immune system lets the criminal go free. Instead of being grateful that he wasn't caught and taking the hint to give up his life of crime, the villain carries on growing and mutating with inevitable and distressing results. This is why the findings from some studies are so exciting, which suggest beneficial bacteria might be able to clear up troublesome cells that might otherwise go on to mutate and become carcinogenic.

What impairs our immunity?

I don't think it's difficult to see why our resistance to illness isn't as strong as it might be. What do you think? Here are some dietary and lifestyle possibilities:

- Far fewer people than ever before know how to cook a healthy meal from scratch and so find themselves relying on pre-prepared products that are often loaded with sugar, salt and additives.

- Sugar, processed fat and other junk figures so heavily in most people's diets these days that they're no longer being properly nourished. As adults, we have the choice as to whether or not we allow ourselves to become addicted to plastic, processed pseudo food. Unfortunately, we're also inflicting what has become a life-threatening habit onto our children, setting them up for a future of obesity, heart disease and premature death. It's been suggested that the effects of this change are so severe and that children are missing out to such a worrying degree on proper nourishment that many parents may, in all probability, outlive their own offspring.

- Along similar lines, population studies suggest that the reluctance to include fresh fruits and vegetables in the diet is leading to borderline nutrient deficiencies across all age groups. In other words, large chunks of the population are not taking enough nourishment from their diets for optimum health.

- Breastfeeding, known for the extra protection it can confer from a healthy mother to a newborn, is too often ousted by formula feeds. Nor do babies receive the extended breastfeeding favoured by previous generations. Experts are concerned that little ones who miss out on this protection early in life may be more susceptible to future illness. Read more about this in Chapter 22.

Caesarean section and lack of mother's milk may therefore contribute to immune system problems. Some formula feeds are now beginning to include probiotics although these can never totally replace the benefits of breastfeeding.

- The majority of babies are weaned on to processed purées. Preparing home-made purée from fresh ingredients seems the exception these days rather than the norm. Yet, generally speaking, processed food is nearly always going to be less nutritious than something made from fresh produce.

- Eczema, asthma and allergy-related illness is more common in bottlefed babies than in breastfed babies. In addition, it's known that colds, influenza, throat and chest infections, common enough in the average population, appear far more frequently and persistently in asthma and allergy sufferers of all ages. In one study, around 80 per cent of mucus samples taken from asthmatic children were found to contain active cold viruses, demonstrating that their immunity is under pressure.

- Clinical experience suggests that immunity may be being affected by a number of prescribed medications. One of the most obvious is antibiotics, which upset the system by disturbing the balance of protective beneficial bacteria.

- Environmental pollution (and 'chemicals with everything') puts further strain on the immune system, as it works ever harder to protect the body from threatening outside influences.

Where do probiotics fit into all this?

Apart from their importance in promoting a healthy gut and fighting the bad guys, research tells us that probiotics are also very much involved in the operation of different immune cells, which protect us against disease, and that taking probiotics enhances our immune response to viral and bacterial infections.

They're also anti-inflammatory (they can help to calm or cancel inflammation). It's our good gut bugs – the resident microflora as well as the probiotics we take in our diets – which play a significant role in maintaining the support of a special battalion of protectors called secretory IgA, or SIgA. Special Agent SIgA helps to defend us against infections such as fungi, viruses and parasites. It's also important for regulating (controlling and calming) the inflammatory processes, which is why imbalances can sometimes be found in diseases that are associated with excess inflammation. Now researchers are trying to find out how friendly flora actually do this. So far, they know that good gut bugs are somehow involved in the development of those special peacekeeping cells – called regulatory T cells – that are in charge of the inflammation OFF switch and possibly also in the messaging system that exists between certain immune cells. Probiotics could also play a part in producing antibodies, which may help to reduce the way someone reacts – or overreacts – to an allergen, such as pollen, mould or house-dust mite. Having the right amount of beneficial bacteria not only gives vital support to different areas of the immune system but it can also help the body to eliminate cancer-causing toxins, too. And by helping with oestrogen balance the good gut bacteria could also be important in helping to protect us from certain hormonal cancers.

It's hardly any wonder, then, that the use of good bacteria as a possible catalyst to boost immunity is now so much in the spotlight.

Part Three

Supplements and Safety

25.

Choosing Probiotic Foods and Supplements

'Many commercially driven probiotics remain big hitters in the
alternative medicine arena. In contrast to many inhabitants of the
fringe scene, they do however have a record of properly
conducted trials confirming efficacy in specific areas notably
infectious diarrhoea and urogenital infections and a burgeoning
portfolio of basic scientific studies . . . No other therapeutic
modality spans the divide between Internet voodoo and
cutting-edge high-tech in this way. '

Simon H. Murch, 'Probiotics as mainstream allergy therapy?', commentary in the
peer review journal, *Archives of Diseases in Childhood* 2005;90:881–2

When shopping for probiotics, it's important to understand that
as well as being available in a wide variety of guises – as
capsules, tablets or powders – there are also huge differences in
strength and quality. Not all products are equal: some are extremely
effective whereas, at the other end of the scale, others simply don't
pass muster. A few are even fake, and a small percentage have
actually been described as 'a pile of poo', because they were found
to contain untested or potentially unsafe faecal or soil organisms.
It's a minefield of microflora out there, so here are some guidelines
to help you avoid the crap trap:

Quality definitely matters

Anything that simply says that it's probiotic without providing any detail is definitely one to avoid. And it doesn't always follow that, because it 'contains beneficial bacteria' or says 'acidophilus' or 'bifidus' on the label, it's going to be helpful. If the product doesn't say how many billion live bacteria are included, or you can't find their names, don't buy it. According to independent surveys, some are either completely conked out well before the bottle is opened or simply don't survive past the expected use-by date.

What you need to look for when buying supplements

- Buy a recognised brand (see Resources).
- Check that it's well within the expiry date.
- Look for familiar types of bacteria such as *Lactobacillus acidophilus* and *Bifidobacterium bifidum*.
- Steer clear of anything containing fewer than 1 billion live cells. But go for bigger doses of 10 or 20 billion if you're taking them with or after antibiotics.
- If you need the supplements for travelling, check they don't need to be kept in the fridge.

Now read on to find out more.

Beware of unconvincing wording

If you pick up a product where the labelling seems excessive or the wording unconvincing, then it probably isn't the real deal; for example, under both UK and European Union law anything claiming that it can prevent, treat or cure a condition or vague notions that something might 'help your body to resist stress' is a no-no, as is any inference that a brand or ingredient has been endorsed by a doctor or other health professional.

This doesn't mean that products without official declarations are bad for you. In the United Kingdom, at the time of writing, you won't find any health benefits or pronouncements shown on supplement labels (and that includes probiotics), because they all come under the category of foods, not medicines, and to link a food product to a medicinal effect isn't legal. It's important to keep in mind, however, that labelling legislation is an ongoing process and things are changing all the time.

What matters most is that any info about nutritional or health benefits in either food or food supplements has to be truthful, clear, accurate and meaningful, should not mislead the consumer and must be able to be substantiated. The onus is on the supplement supplier to provide as much information as possible and also to prove that any given probiotic strain is safe. Reliable companies will usually provide contact details so that you can get in touch should you need more info. Good manufacturers who have high standards and know the law won't try to pull the wool over your eyes.

What's the deal on dosage?

Good-quality probiotic products will tell you on the label the type of bacteria they contain as well as (very important) the potency. Dosages aren't expressed in grams or milligrams as they are in most other supplements. Most probiotics are measured in millions or billions of microorganisms or live cells, known as the viability count. Sometimes, in the literature or on the labelling, you might see the letters CFU, which stand for colony forming units, the system of measurement used to calculate viable (live) bacteria. If a supplement has fewer than 10 million then it's generally considered not to be worthwhile. In fact, in the vast ocean of your intestines, 10 million bacteria are, quite literally, a microscopic drop.

Remember that if your product contains more than one type of bacteria, the label will either give you an overall total of the number of friendly flora or the individual quantity alongside each of the different strains, in which case you will need to add them up. So it might say *Lactobacillus acidophilus* 1 billion, *Bifidobacterium bifidum* 1 billion and *Lactobacillus rhamnosus* GG 1 billion, which means you have a probiotic supplement containing 3 billion organisms.

While most suppliers will state the number of organisms on the label, remember that independent testing has shown that several products have fallen short of their claimed targets. That's why it is so important to (a) buy a recognised brand; and (b) to make sure it's well within date. On some brands, you may still see the phrase 'at the time of manufacture' indicating the bacterial count when the product was packaged. This reference is gradually being phased out and, before too long, best practice recommendations should have brought about a change of wording so that, instead, all products will tell you the likely potency at the expiry date.

What you should get in a good product

Although you won't know this from reading the label, you can be confident that reliable producers of probiotics will ensure that the bacteria in your supplement:

- Have a history of safe use, are non-toxic and non-pathogenic.
- Are alive and kicking when administered.
- Are stable and will survive storage for the life of the product.
- In the case of probiotics that are used for vaginal treatment, are tough enough to resist spermicides.

Should probiotics be refrigerated?

When you buy, look for information on how best to store the product. Some require refrigeration and some don't, but in any case keeping the product in the fridge will always extend its shelf life. Those that survive outside the fridge are useful if you're away from home and want to take your supplements with you.

Be guided by price

One of the best guides to quality is price. Although it's a frequent groan that most probiotics are expensive, you do tend to get what you pay for. This is because good manufacturing practice, extensive research and development, the latest production techniques, effective ingredients and protective, properly vacuum-sealed packaging all cost money.

When you first start

If you begin a course of probiotics and find you're suffering a grumble of gas in the nether regions, this doesn't mean that what you are taking is bad for you or causing you any harm. Very occasionally, when a person alters and improves their diet, they might find flatulence, abdominal bloating, headaches or changes in their bowel habit. The same thing can happen when you introduce good gut bugs into the system. Even though it may seem like a backward step, it's nearly always a positive sign that everything is working as it should. Something similar is known as the Jarisch-Herxheimer reaction, named after the German doctor who first noticed it. The most severe type of 'Herx' occurs when, as a result of swathes of bad yeasts and pathogens dying off following antibiotic therapy, large quantities of toxins are released into the bloodstream. The unpleasant symptoms are a consequence of those toxins being produced faster than the liver or kidneys can deal with them. The phenomenon of things appearing to get worse before they get better is also sometimes called a healing crisis.

The reaction occurs as the system begins to discard waste. When you suddenly introduce helpful bacteria into your intestines, your exit routes can become congested with pathogenic bacteria and toxins that are being bumped off in great numbers. Don't be concerned. Any symptoms should only be temporary. Remember that the level of any reaction will depend entirely upon your level of tolerance and you may notice absolutely no symptoms at all.

If you're affected, the best advice is to cut the supplements out for a couple of days and then begin again with the lowest possible dose. Even if the pack advises you to take one or two tablets or capsules per day, ignore this for the moment and take one every other day for a week. Then over the next few days increase to the recommended dose.

It can also help if you drink plenty of water. This increases the blood volume and encourages flushing out of the kidneys.

Why not just eat yoghurt?

Supermarket shelves are groaning under the weight of an incredible array of 'smart' dairy foods. But do they all live up to their claims? Are they really helpful? And are they a good enough substitute for probiotic supplements?

Some yoghurt and yoghurt drinks can be a valuable source of probiotic bacteria, but most don't have large amounts. Just bear in mind that there's a big difference between what we call a maintenance dose of live culture in a fresh yoghurt product and the therapeutic levels that can be found in a quality probiotic supplement. However, that doesn't mean the beneficial bacteria in foods aren't useful. They're certainly good to take on a day-to-day basis and can provide valuable extra nourishment. The problem lies in what to choose.

Occasional reports have suggested that there aren't enough friendly bacteria in yoghurt products able to survive the stomach acid or to have any helpful impact on the intestines. Although what you will find in a good probiotic drink or yoghurt isn't much when compared to a quality supplement, the vast majority of strains that are used in these food products are acid tolerant and are therefore likely to survive their intestinal journey. There's also evidence in the medical literature that live yoghurt and probiotic shots can help to reduce the side effects of antibiotics, especially diarrhoea.

However, if you're dealing with a health problem or have had digestive or bowel troubles for some time, then a one-a-day yoghurt or probiotic drink may not have quite enough oomph and won't always be sufficient to redress the balance where gut flora is seriously disturbed.

A major downside of many yoghurts and yoghurt drinks is that the sugar content can be quite high, making the vast majority of them out of bounds for diabetics, for people suffering candida yeast infections, those battling obesity or folks who are just trying to avoid sugar. I think it would be a positive move by the manufacturers if they were to reduce the sugar levels without resorting to artificial sweeteners, especially as they continually promote their products as being healthy.

Shopping guide for yoghurt products

- Scrutinise the labels. In particular, they should tell you whether or not there is any live culture. Look out for words such as 'fermented' or Latin names like *Lactobacillus acidophilus, L. bulgaricus* or *L. casei*.

- Make sure that the yoghurt or yoghurt drink is well within the use-by date and allow for the fact that it may be even nearer the date by the time you get to consume it. If it's already close to expiry, then don't buy it.

- Take an insulated 'cold' bag or box with you to transport chilled foods and put them straight into the refrigerator when you get home.

- Be wary of anything claiming to be 'sugar-free'. They usually contain artificial sweeteners, and chemical sweeteners can actually encourage you to crave carbohydrates. Manufacturers do also sometimes say 'sucrose-free', giving the impression that it has no sugar, but then incorporate maltose, dextrose or glucose, or the ubiquitous aspartame.

- You'll certainly find that most products claiming to be low calorie or zero fat will have plenty of fairly unnatural-sounding things listed on the label. It's better to buy the unadulterated full-fat version (see page 55) and eat less of it than to load your body with a cocktail of questionable chemicals.

- Why not just go for plain, additive-free, yoghurt? If you have a really sweet tooth, stir in a small quantity of quality honey, which is naturally prebiotic. (If you're dealing with *Helicobacter pylori* or any kind of infection, then I would very strongly recommend that you invest in a jar of high-strength Comvita Manuka Honey – see Resources.)

- If cow's milk is a problem food for you, try yoghurts made from goat's or sheep's milk. You can find them in some supermarkets and also in independent health-food stores. Soya yoghurts are also available, although they do not suit everybody. And bear in mind that, unless you suffer from a classical acute allergic reaction to dairy protein, fermented foods such as kefir and buttermilk may be easier to digest and better for your health than straight cow's milk.

These foods are certainly a worthwhile option for anyone with lactose intolerance (see page 218).

Any more questions?

Check out the FAQs in Chapter 26 and also pages 121–2 in Chapter 7.

26.

FAQs about Probiotics

Q: Should I take probiotics all the time?

A: Although regular use is recommended, it doesn't necessarily mean that you need to take probiotic supplements every single day. The important thing is to try to ensure frequent top-ups.

The reason for this is because these helpful microorganisms are washed out within a few weeks. It's worth emphasising here that if the resident bacteria (the locals) have been damaged or depleted in the gut, not only are the probiotics you swallow going to be involved in repopulating the area but they're also going to make life pretty uncomfortable for any pathogenic hangers-on such as bad bacteria, parasites and yeasts.

Start with a course of, say, two or three months and continue for longer than that if you've been suffering with a particularly difficult gut problem or recurring bouts of any of the illnesses I've discussed in Part Two. After that, take a repeat course whenever you can afford it, certainly every few months – as well as during and after any antibiotic treatment. Another option would be to follow the initial course as suggested above, and then after that take your probiotics every other day. This means that a normal pack scheduled to last one month will, in fact, stretch to two months, thereby keeping costs down.

Q: How much should I take?

A: Opinions vary widely as to the optimum for an actual supplement. Some experts suggest 3, 5, 10 or 20 billion whereas others say that 1 billion is plenty. In the future, as more clinical studies link particular strains of probiotic to particular health benefits, it's expected that manufacturers will be able to develop products that target specific conditions. In the meantime, since research suggests that more is better – especially when using after antibiotics – I would go for something with a larger amount for at least the first month and then reduce to a lower maintenance dose.

Q: If I'm taking antibiotics, when should I introduce probiotics?

A: The best advice is to start a course of probiotics in tandem with the antibiotics and then continue taking the probiotics for a while after the antibiotics are finished. Chapter 7 on antibiotics (page 121) has detailed information on this point. The most important thing to remember is to always take a course of probiotics if you have had to have antibiotics.

Q: For how long should I take probiotics?

A: The length of time required to repopulate the gut will depend on several factors including the quality of the product you choose, the type of bacteria it contains and your general health status. How much beneficial bacteria you need to consume may also be affected by how long you've had the symptoms and your general health before this particular episode of bad health occurred. If you're suffering from candidiasis or leaky gut syndrome, for example, or your gut has been devastated by multiple courses of antibiotics, you might benefit from a much longer course of several months. If colds and respiratory infections are your main problem, taking probiotics every day for three months during the winter could be valuable. You may even be advised by your practitioner to add them permanently to your daily routine.

Q: Is the use-by date really that important?

A: Very important indeed. Always buy well within date. The number of bacteria in a product at the time of manufacture and distribution will nearly always dwindle naturally during storage, but products way past their date will probably have few, if any, active bacteria. Reliable producers of probiotics will usually put in more bacteria than it says on the label.

Q: Sometimes there are numbers or letters written after the Latin name. What do these mean?

A: These indicate the strain of a particular bacterium.

> **Names and strains**
> When we talk about probiotic bacteria, we use the Latin, for example, *Lactobacillus acidophilus*. The first part of the name is called the genus. So other bacteria labelled *Lactobacillus*, such as *Lactobacillus reuteri* or *L. casei*, are closely related and belong to the same large family. The second half, *acidophilus*, is a bit like someone's surname and indicates the particular species or relative in that family. Any extra letters or numbers signify the specific strain of a bacteria as in *Lactobacillus rhamnosus* GG or *Streptococcus salivarius* K12, and are equivalent to a person's first name.

Q: Which bacteria should I look for?

A: Some of the products you see for sale will contain only a single type of bacterium (commonly *Lactobacillus acidophilus*) but most will include more than one. If you're still unsure, I suggest that your probiotic supplement contains at least *Lactobacillus acidophilus* and *Bifidobacterium*. Both these bacteria withstand acidic conditions and so are more likely to make it through the stomach. They have a history of safe use and there are many scientific studies to back up commonly used strains.

Latin on the label

These are just some of the species of beneficial bacteria that you might see listed on product packaging:

Lactobacillus acidophilus
Lactobacillus brevis
Lactobacillus casei
Lactobacillus delbrueckii (also known as *Lactobacillus bulgaricus*)
Lactobacillus helveticus
Lactobacillus kefir
Lactobacillus lactis
Lactobacillus paracasei
Lactobacillus plantarum
Lactobacillus reuteri
Lactobacillus rhamnosus
Bifidobacterium animalis
Bifidobacterium bifidum
Bifidobacterium infantis
Bifidobacterium lactis
Bifidobacterium longum
Streptococcus thermophilus

Lactobacillus rhamnosus GG is also widely researched. So are *Bifidobacterium lactis* and *L. delbrueckii* (*L. bulgaricus*); the latter is often used as a starter culture for yoghurt products.

Q: Is there any likelihood of probiotics upsetting my existing medication?

A: It's not likely, but as a precaution, it's best not to swallow probiotics in the same mouthful as prescription drugs. In fact, it's always wise to take any kind of supplement, including probiotics, at a different time of day to regular prescribed or over-the-counter medicines. It may be worth mentioning here that, in practice, I've used probiotics very successfully in patients who are taking immune-suppressing medication, but this should only ever be done under medical supervision.

Q: I've been looking on the Internet at some of the research into probiotics. Why are there such varying results?

A: There will always be conflict when it comes to scientific studies. One group of researchers may look at a product or a nutrient or a drug and get startlingly good results, and then another team can come along and do a different study that shows the opposite. Sometimes, scientists might begin with the intention of proving a particular point and end up with an opposite opinion. Results from animal studies may differ considerably from those on humans even if the type of probiotic used is the same. Different doses of the same probiotic can produce entirely different results, as can different strains of the same family of bacteria. The outcome may also be affected by how the probiotic was administered during the study (by mouth or intravenously, and so on).

Differences are accepted as inevitable, especially in clinical trials using human subjects. Every person involved will have an individual health status and history, and doctors now think that even someone's natural biological and physiological cycle could affect the outcome.

Q: Are probiotics safe?

A: The commonly used strains are deemed to be incredibly safe and, overall, there have been no serious safety issues with regard to either probiotic supplements or drinks. If there were going to be problems, it would be natural to expect some kind of corresponding increase in adverse reactions in consumers to match the massive boom in the use of well-known types of friendly flora. This hasn't happened. In fact, there is growing evidence to show that the familiar species can be used without any threat of interference to existing medication or diet. In an assessment made by a prestigious group of some of the world's leading probiotic experts and researchers, the likelihood of any infection being caused by the consumption of *Lactobacillus acidophilus* and *Bifidobacterium* was considered to be 'negligible'.

There have been a handful of reports where products containing soil organisms, a very dodgy one in particular called *Bacillus subtilis*, caused severe problems, including septicaemia. This isn't surprising since soil-borne bacteria are not part of the normal microflora of a human gut. It's unlikely now that you will come across any product containing *Bacillus subtilis* but if you do, don't buy it.

There have also been headlined press reports concerning some patients with a serious condition known as pancreatitis who died after they were given something that was reported as being a probiotic. However, this needs to be seen in context. It was a product that didn't meet the 'minimum criteria to properly be called a probiotic'. Furthermore, there were no published data to show that it was either safe or beneficial to use. Nor did it give details of the strain or type of bacteria. The people concerned were already very sick indeed; also the mortality was not due to infections caused by the product but by multiple organ failure. This is a classic example of conclusions and assumptions being made in the wake of just one uncommon and isolated case.

In another study of patients suffering severe pancreatitis, treatment using *Lactobacillus plantarum* 299V showed a significant decrease in infection. See what I mean about there always being opposing findings in scientific studies?

For everyone else, probiotics offer a very safe option. Even really poorly patients can benefit. In a controlled clinical trial of patients undergoing liver transplant, where several strains of probiotics were given alongside prebiotic fibre, only one patient out of 33 contracted a post-operative infection compared to 17 out of 33 in the control group who received no supplements. Other research showed that giving probiotics to some critically ill patients actually helped to *prevent* multiple organ failure. And in a study of people who were HIV-positive, they were found to tolerate a daily dose of 10 billion *Lactobacillus reuteri* with no adverse reaction or safety issues.

> **A record of safety**
> 'Given that an estimated 20 billion doses of probiotics are consumed each year, with only four cases of bacteremia [bacteria in the blood] associated with their use over the past 10 years, probiotic therapy is significantly safer than pharmaceutical agents.'
> Dr Gregor Reid, 'The importance of guidelines in the development and application of probiotics', *Current Pharmaceutical Design*, 2005;11:11–16

Q: When should I not take probiotics?

A: There are a handful of situations where probiotics may not be appropriate. As a precaution I would advise that probiotic supplements are not used in transplant patients nor in anyone who is undergoing abdominal surgery, has ruptured intestinal tissue, perforation of the bowel or is in intensive care, unless supervised by a specialist. In other cases of serious ill-health, such as cancer or disorders of the immune system, or anyone who is on immune-suppressant medication, always talk to the doctor or consultant in charge of your case. If you have any serious illness such as pancreatitis or damage to the bowel wall then, again, don't take probiotics without the support, approval and regular monitoring of your medical or surgical adviser.

There are a few reports that suggest probiotics are not suitable in cases of IBD (inflammatory bowel disease) such as Crohn's or ulcerative colitis, but there are also a number of studies demonstrating how helpful they can be. In my practice I have found probiotics to be extremely beneficial, but the best advice would be to use them *only* if you are under the care of a qualified nutritionist or health-care provider who has extensive experience using probiotic therapy.

Q: I bought a probiotic product and then read the label, which said it contained yeast. I thought yeast was a bad thing.

A: There are some kinds of beneficial yeasts (not to be confused with candida yeast) that have a probiotic action and are therefore sometimes included in probiotic supplements. Probably the best known of these is *Saccharomyces boulardii* (now called *Saccharomyces cerevisiae*), which has been extensively researched and shown to be helpful in a range of different conditions. However, there have been a few reported cases of a fungal infection of the blood known as fungaemia which occurred in patients fitted with intravenous catheters who were also taking this probiotic yeast. Although fungaemia is something that is really only likely to occur in seriously ill patients, such as those in intensive care or following extensive antibiotic therapy, I think it's wise to be cautious and to leave *S. cerevisiae* for medical use only.

Q: I saw the letters FOS on the label. What does this stands for?

A: FOS is a fructo-oligosaccharide (see page 78 of Chapter 4). It's a prebiotic, not a probiotic, but is often included in probiotic supplements. Studies show that FOS can be a helpful addition to the diet, which is why it's sometimes recommended to diabetics as an alternative to sugar or sweeteners. However, it may not be suitable for a digestive system that is particularly sensitive.

If your gut is under the weather and your system is lacking in beneficial bacteria, FOS can sometimes cause flatulence. However, whether you are using a dedicated FOS product or are taking it as part of your probiotic supplement, the gassy side effects can be overcome by starting off with a very low dose and working up to the recommended intake over a period of weeks. If you suffer with irritable bowel syndrome, see my note about FOS in that chapter.

Q: How and when should I take my supplements?

A: Always follow the pack instructions. Some probiotics state 'between meals' and others 'with food'. Heat destroys probiotics, so avoid swallowing them with a hot drink or hot food. Most types of probiotic do appreciate a bit of food to help them on their journey because this tends to protect them from the ravages of the stomach acid. So you might take them with a drink of water just before you sit down to a meal (any time of day is fine but see my note on page 121 concerning how to use probiotics when you're using antibiotics). Or take your probiotic immediately before breakfast with a glass of water, together with milled flax fibre or psyllium husk powder (see page 99). Then eat your breakfast. If your particular product recommends multiple doses (several times a day), then just before meals is probably the best time.

A final word

Always remember that there are many things in everyday life – apart from courses of antibiotics – that can continually damage or disturb the bacterial balance of your body. Excessive stress, ill-health, other prescription medicines, antibiotic residues in food, cigarette smoke, and a not-so-great diet are just a few examples. That's why it makes sense to give yourself regular replenishing treatments to make sure that you discourage harmful pathogens, bacteria and yeasts from setting up home in your gut, and to help support your immune system.

27.

Resources

Contact individual companies or search their websites for more information. If you don't have access to the Internet or prefer not to shop online, quite a few of the products mentioned are available from department stores, major supermarkets and smaller independent stores throughout the UK.

At-a-glance product search

Check main list for contact details.

Aloe 99 gel Xynergy Health Products
Bleach-free sanitary protection Natracare
Coenzyme Q$_{10}$ Pharma Nord
Comvita Manuka Honey Xynergy Health Products
E-cloths Enviro Products, Lakeland Limited
Eco skin care/body care Lucy Russell Organics, Green People, Xynergy Health Products, Victoria Health, Beauty Bazaar, Big Green Smile
Fibre supplements Nutrigold, Biocare, G&G Foods, Victoria Health, Solgar, Higher Nature, Arkopharma
Glyconutrients for urinary and other health problems Sweet Cures of York
Goat's milk formula Nanny Care
Herbal medicines Arkopharma, Natural Dispensary, Sunshine Health Shop, Biocare, Viridian Nutrition, Solgar, Victoria Health, Nutri Centre
Household cleaning Method, Bio-D Company, Ecozone, Enviro Products, Ecover, Natural Collection, Big Green Smile

Natural toothpaste, mouthwash Green People, Xynergy Health Products

Probiotics Supplements Natural Dispensary, Sunshine Health Shop, Victoria Health, Biocare, Viridian Nutrition, Solgar, Lamberts, Nature's Best, Nutri Centre, G&G

Probiotics for oral health Blis Technologies

Vitamin and mineral supplements/antioxidants Biocare, Pharma Nord, Solgar, Lamberts, Nature's Best, Natural Dispensary, Sunshine Health Shop, Nutri Centre, Victoria Health, Viridian Nutrition, G&G

Washing and tumble-drying without chemicals Ecozone, Lakeland Limited

Suppliers' contact details

Arkopharma, www.arkopharma.com
Arkocaps herbal medicines. Also available from The Nutri Centre, health stores and some pharmacies

Beauty Bazaar, www.beautybazaar.co.uk
customerservice@beautybazaar.co.uk
Telephone: 0800 027 1102
Skin and body care. For high-street stockists of skin-care brands Logona, Sante, Santaverde, La Clarée, Florascent, Amber Gel and Huiles & Baumes, contact www.avea.co.uk

Big Green Smile, www.biggreensmile.com
Telephone: 0845 230 2365
Supplier of Avalon organics and a wide range of eco-friendly products, including Bentley and Quash

Biocare, www.biocare.co.uk
Vitamin C 500 & 1000 magnesium ascorbate, broad-spectrum amino acids, Intrafresh pessaries for vaginal use, probiotics including those suitable for babies and young children, strawberry and banana flavoured probiotics, *Bifidobacterium infantis*, cranberry complex, multivitamin/mineral complexes, liquid vitamin and mineral preparations

Bio-D Company, www.biodegradable.biz
Eco-friendly household cleaning products

Bioforce, www.bioforceshop.co.uk
Telephone helpline: 0845 608 5858
Dr Vogel Echinaforce tincture and tablets, Molkosan, uva-ursi tincture, natural deodorant, neem oil products, herbal remedies for sleep and relaxation

Bionutri products are available from:
Sunshine Health Shop, www.sunshinehealthshop.co.uk
Telephone: 01453 751395
Natural Dispensary, see below
The Nutri Centre, see below
Revital, www.revital.co.uk
Telephone: 0870 366 5729
Elderberry complex, junior elderberry, vitamin C complex, probiotic ecodophilus, cardiomega, Estrolignan

Blis Technologies, Centre for Innovation, University of Otago, Dunedin, New Zealand, www.blis.co.nz
Streptococcus salivarius K12, throat lozenges and dental packages for oral health and halitosis. Products available in several countries under different brand names (contact Blis for further information)

Blue Herbs, www.blueherbs.co.uk, www.blessedherbs.com
Herbal products for colon cleansing and parasite removal. Expensive but effective

Dietary Needs Direct, www.dietaryneedsdirect.co.uk
Telephone: 01453 790 999
Products for people who prefer to avoid wheat and dairy

Dr Vogel, www.avogel.co.uk
Telephone: 0845 608 5858
Dr Vogel Echinaforce tincture and tablets

Enviro Products Ltd, www.e-cloth.com
Telephone: 01892 752199
E-cloth system. Range of cleaning cloths and mops which work without household chemicals. Especially good if you suffer from

allergies or prefer to avoid using chemical cleaning products.
Available by mail from the manufacturer and from Lakeland
Limited, www.lakelandlimited.co.uk, telephone: 015394 88100

Ecozone, www.ecozone.co.uk
Telephone: 0208 662 7222
Specialists in eco-friendly products, including Eco-balls for machine
washing without soap. Also stockists for Green People and Biocare

G&G Foods, www.gandginfo.com
Fibre Detox powder, GC70 fibre cleansing pack, Natren brand
probiotics, G&G brand probiotics, anti-parasitic herbal preparations

Genova Diagnostics, www.gdx.uk.net
infouk@gdx.net
Telephone: 0208 336 7750
Wide ranging diagnostic tests for allergies, candidiasis, etc

Green People, www.greenpeople.co.uk
Fennel & Propolis Toothpaste, Fennel Mouthwash, Antibacterial
Handwash, Foaming Hand Sanitizer, 'No Scent' Deodorant

Lakeland Limited, www.lakelandlimited.co.uk
Telephone: 015394 88100
Online and from Lakeland stores: E cloths: Microfibre cloths that
clean without the need for soap or detergents, and washing and
tumble-drying products that reduce or avoid the use of detergent
soaps and fabric softener

Lamberts Healthcare, 1 Lamberts Road, Tunbridge Wells, Kent
TN2 3EH
Telephone: 01892 554312
Wide range of supplements including probiotics. Practitioner
supply only

Laundry Labs, www.laundrylabs.com
info@thelaundrylabs.com
Telephone: 0845 872 4955
Tumble Dryerballs – avoids the need for fabric softener

Lucy Russell Organics, www.lucyrussellorganics.co.uk
info@lucyrussellorganics.co.uk

Lucy Russell Organics *cont.*, Telephone: 0845 094 2227
Organic skin care

Method, www.methodhome.com
talkclean@methodhome.com
Telephone: 0207 788 7904
Eco-friendly household cleaning products. Products available from major supermarkets and department stores and smaller independents, online and throughout the UK

Nature's Best, Century Place, Tunbridge Wells, Kent TN2 3BE
www.naturesbest.co.uk
info@naturesbest.co.uk
Telephone, order line: 01892 552 117
Wide range of vitamins, minerals, omega-3 supplements and probiotics

The Natural Dispensary, 26 Church Street, Stroud,
Gloucestershire GL5 1JL
www.naturaldispensary.com
Telephone: 01453 757792
One-stop shop for best-quality supplements including Biocare, Bionutri, Dr Vogel, Lamberts, Solgar, Viridian Nutrition. The Natural Dispensary will send products UK-wide and overseas

Natracare, www.natracare.com
Telephone: 0117 982 3492
One-hundred per cent organic cotton sanitary protection including pads, towels, tampons and intimate wipes, also baby wipes. All biodegradable and free from chlorine, sodium laurel sulphate, parabens and perfumes

Nutrigold Colon Support Formula is available from:
Natural Dispensary, see above; Sunshine Health Shop, see Bionutri; Victoria Health, see below; Nutri Centre, see the next page

Nanny Care, www.vitacare.co.uk
enquiry@vitacare.co.uk
NannyCare formula and other goat's milk products

Natural Collection, www.naturalcollection.com
enquiries@naturalcollection.com

Telephone: 0845 367 7001
Also at Ethical Superstore,
enquiries@ethicalsuperstore.com
Telephone: 0800 999 2134
Eco-friendly household cleaning

Nutri Centre, www.NutriCentre.com
Go to website for store locator
Vitamin/mineral supplements, probiotics, herbal medicines,
natural skin-care products

Pharma Nord UK, www.pharmanord.co.uk
Telephone: 01670 519989
Bio-quinone 100mg, Bio-quinone 30mg

Solgar, www.solgar.com
Telephone: 01442 890355
Advanced Acidophilus range, Multiacidophilus powder, Olive Leaf
Echinacea Complex, Psyllium Husk Fibre, multivitamin/mineral
supplements

Sunshine Health Shop, www.sunshinehealthshop.co.uk
Telephone: 01453 763 923
Quality supplements and health foods despatched to the UK and
worldwide. Also owns Dietary Needs Direct

Sweet Cures of York, www.sweetcures.com
Telephone: 01904 789559
Glyconutrients
D-mannose, Xylotene
Other useful links:
www.Waterfall-D-Mannose.com; www.urologyadvice.com;
www.cystitis-cystitis.com/research.htm

Victoria Health, www.victoriahealth.com
Telephone: 0800 3898195
Wide range of supplements, probiotics, herbals, skin-care and
body-care products

Viridian Nutrition, 31 Alvis Way, Royal Oak, Daventry, Northamptonshire NN11 8PG
www.viridian-nutrition.com
Telephone: 01327 878050
Viridian Cranberry, Viridian Ester-C, probiotics for children and adults, excellent multivitamin products, range of herbals, 100% Organic Golden Flaxseed Oil

York Laboratories, www.yorktest.com
Telephone: 01904 410410
Allergy testing

Xynergy Health Products, www.xynergy.co.uk
Telephone: 08456 585858
UMF 15+ Comvita Manuka Honey, UMF 20+, UMF 25+, Comvita Toothgel, Comvita Propolis Soap, Kiwiherb Mouthwash, Neem Mouthwash, Propolis Soap, Propolis Throat Spray, Natural Deodorant Crystal, Comvita Olive Leaf Complex

---

Information on candida

The National Candida Society is an experienced support group. They send out a very good quarterly newsletter or e-letter and have a helpline. There are 40+ local support groups across the UK. Being part of a group of people experiencing similar difficulties can be rewarding and may be helpful for your own recovery. Website www.candida-society.org.uk.

The Practical Guide To Candida by Jane McWhirter contains much valuable help on the condition of candidiasis. It costs £11 from the Nutri Centre bookshop, telephone 0207 323 2382, or direct from Jane Lorimer, Gibliston Mill, Colinsburgh, Leven, Fife KY9 1JS. You might also be interested in Jane's DVD, *Clear From Candida*. It's comprehensive and detailed with a three-hour running time, including an hour's cooking demonstration. Cost is £21 including the recipe booklet.

In addition to the above, the following website has useful information: www.cgstock.com/candida/research/html

Afterword

I first met Kathryn Marsden in 2007 at the home of a mutual friend. When the conversation got around to people's ailments – as it tends to do when you're all over a certain age – I found out that she was a nutritionist. I have very high cholesterol but am allergic to statins (cholesterol-lowering drugs) and in my quest to stay healthy without medication I've done a lot of reading about diet and food supplements. Within a few minutes of talking to Kathryn I realised that I was in the company of someone who really knew her subject. She was also unassuming and genuinely interested in helping people improve their lives. I later looked her up on the Internet and discovered that she is the author of several successful books on the subject of health and that one of her special interests was the dietary treatment of gut ailments. It got me wondering if she could help my daughter Susannah.

Susannah had been suffering from bouts of severe stomach and abdominal pain for several years and these were becoming quite debilitating. She had seen several doctors and hospital specialists who concluded that she had irritable bowel syndrome, probably triggered by stress. Susannah had tried all the usual treatments for this condition but without success.

An appointment was arranged and Kathryn made a full evaluation of Susannah's symptoms. At the end of a very thorough discussion, she concluded that Susannah's condition was likely being caused or aggravated by three major problems: an allergy to wheat; a low intake of fluid; and disturbed gut flora. She did not believe that Susannah had IBS since, apart from gut pain, there were none of the other symptoms that are typical of the condition. Kathryn suggested that Susannah avoid all wheat-based foods, particularly bread and bran cereals, introduce alternative sources of fibre, drink more water and take a course of probiotic supplements.

Susannah was a little sceptical but introduced Kathryn's recommendations. It has changed her life. She has not had a single episode of stomach or gut pain since that time. As a result of feeling so much better, Susannah's career has reached new heights, which would not have been possible in the state she was in before. We are so grateful to Kathryn. This woman definitely knows her stuff.

Richard Perry
Teulada,
Spain

Sources of Reference

The author fully acknowledges the work of the many experts working in the field of probiotics and prebiotics. To obtain material for this project, Kathryn referred to more than 700 different documents. To save both paper and space she has listed only a small number of key references here. The full list is available online at www.goodgutbugs.weebly.com

Part One

'Inspection of cleanliness and infection control: How well are acute trusts following the hygiene code?' *Report of the UK Healthcare Commission* 24 November 2008.
'Maggots help cure MRSA patients', BBC News, 2 May 2007. http://news.bbc.co.uk/2/hi/uk_news/england/manchester/6614471.stm; 'Red Army virus to combat MRSA', BBC News, 13 August 2007, http://news.bbc.co.uk/2/hi/health/6943779.stm
UK Office for National Statistics, 'Deaths involving *Clostridium difficile* by communal establishment, England and Wales 2007'. Posted 28 August 2008, www.statistics.gov.uk; 'Improving patient care by reducing the risk of hospital acquired infection: A progress report', TSO The Stationery Office 14 July 2004 ISBN 9780 102929157; The Association for Professionals in Infection Control and Epidemiology, 'Guidelines for the Control of MRSA', June 2008

Andoh A., et al., 'Role of dietary fiber and short-chain fatty acids in the colon', *Current Pharmaceutical Design* 2003;9(4):347–58.
Aslam S., et al., 'Treatment of *Clostridium difficile*-associated disease: Old therapies and new strategies', *Lancet Infectious Diseases* 2005;5:549–57.
Bagchi D. and Dash S.K., '*Lactobacillus acidophilus*: Natural antibiotics and beyond', *Townsend Letter for Doctors and Patients* 1996;77–82.
Baker R., 'Health management with reduced antibiotic use: The U.S. experience', *Animal Biotechnology* 2006;17(2):195–205.
Bartlett J.G., 'Narrative review: The new epidemic of *Clostridium difficile*-associated enteric disease', *Annals of Internal Medicine* 2006;145:758–64.
Beaugerie L. and Petit J.C., 'Microbial-gut interactions in health and disease: Antibiotic-associated diarrhoea', Review, *Clinical Gastroenterology* 2004; 18(2):337–52.
Blossom D.B. and McDonald L.C., 'The challenges posed by reemerging *Clostridium difficile* infection', *Clinical Infectious Diseases* 2007;45:222–7.
Bronzwaer S., et al., 'European Antimicrobial Resistance Surveillance System (EARSS): Objectives and organisation', *Eurosurveillance* 1999;4(4):41–4.

Callaway, E., 'Superbug "condom" could slow spread of drug resistance', *New Scientist* 19 December 2008; issue 2687.

Carman R.J., et al., 'Ciprofloxacin at low levels disrupts colonization resistance of human fecal microflora growing in chemostats', extract, *Regulatory Toxicology and Pharmacology* 2004;40(3):319–26.

Cherbut C., et al., 'Acacia Gum is a bifidogenic dietary fibre with high digestive tolerance in healthy humans', *Journal of Microbial Ecology in Health and Disease* 2003;15(1):43–50.

Coia J.E., et al., 'Guidelines for the control and prevention of methicillin-resistant *Staphylococcus aureus* (MRSA) in healthcare facilities', *Journal of Hospital Infection* 2006;63(1):S1–44.

Cremonini F., et al., 'Meta-analysis: The effect of probiotic administration on antibiotic-associated diarrhoea', *Alimentary Pharmacology Therapy* 2002; 16:1461–7.

Cummings J.H., et al., 'Prebiotic digestion and fermentation', *American Journal of Clinical Nutrition* 2001;73(2):415S–20S.

Cunnane S.C., et al., 'Nutritional attributes of traditional flaxseed in healthy young adults', *American Journal of Clinical Nutrition* 1995;61:62–8.

EARSS Management Team. Report on feasibility phase EARSS, period: April 1998–September 1999, Bilthoven: RIVM, 1999. http://www.earss.rivm.nl

Floch M.H. and Montrose D.C., 'Use of probiotics in humans: An analysis of the literature', *Gastroenterology Clinics of North America* 2005;34:547–70.

Food and Agriculture Organization of the United Nations (FAO) and the Food Quality and Standards Service (AGNS) Technical Meeting Report. FAO Technical Meeting on PREBIOTICS, 15–16 September 2007. www.fao.org/ag/agn/agns/index_en.stm

Gibson G.R. and Roberfroid M.B., 'Dietary modulation of the human colonic microbiota: Introducing the concept of probiotics', *Journal of Nutrition* 1995;125(6):1401–12.

Gibson G.R., 'Fibre and effects on probiotics (the prebiotic concept)', *Clinical Nutrition Supplements* 2004;1(2):25–31.

Gill H.S. and Guarner F., 'Probiotics and human health: A clinical perspective', *Postgraduate Medical Journal* 2004; 80:516–26.

Guarner F. and Malagelada J.R., 'Gut flora in health and disease', *Lancet* 2003;361(9356):512–19.

Hertzler S.R. and Clancy S.M., 'Kefir improves lactose digestion and tolerance in adults with lactose maldigestion', *Journal of the American Dietetic Association* 2003;103(5):582–7.

Kalser M.H., et al., 'Microflora of the small intestine', *American Journal of Digestive Diseases* 1965;10(10):839–43.

Macfarlane S., et al., 'Prebiotics: Key issues', *Alimentary Pharmacology and Therapeutics* 2006;24:701–14.

Miller G., 'Bestial bugs', *New Scientist* 24 November 2001; issue 2318.

O'Hara A.M. and Shanahan F., 'The gut flora as a forgotten organ', Review, *EMBO Rep.* 2006;7(7):688–93.

O'Sullivan M., 'Probiotic bacteria: Myth or reality?' *Trends in Food Science & Technology* 1992;3:309–14.

Official definition of the word 'probiotic': Joint FAO/WHO Expert Consultation: Report of the Joint Food and Agriculture Organization (FAO) of the United Nations/World Health Organization (WHO) Expert Consultation on Evaluation of Health and Nutritional Properties of Probiotics in Food Including Powder Milk with Live Lactic Acid Bacteria. *Codex Alimentarius Commission* 1–4 October 2001 http://www.who.int/foodsafety/publications/fs_management/en/probiotics.pdf

Pennington, H., 'Don't pick your nose', Letter, *London Review of Books* 15 December 2005;27:24.

Plummer N., et al., 'Fructooligosaccharides and other prebiotics', *Townsend Letter for Doctors and Patients* 2003;239;89–97.

Postgate, J., *Microbes and Man* (fourth edn), Cambridge University Press, 2000.

Reid G., 'The importance of guidelines in the development and application of probiotics', *Current Pharmaceutical Design* 2005;11:11–16.

Reid G., et al., 'Potential uses of probiotics in clinical practice', *Clinical Microbiology Reviews* 2003;16:658–72.

Roberfroid M.B., 'Prebiotics and probiotics: Are they functional foods?', *American Journal of Clinical Nutrition* 2000;71(S):1682S–7S.

Roberfroid M.B., 'Prebiotics: The concept revisited', *Journal of Nutrition* 2007;137:830S–7S.

Saavendra J.M. and Tschemia A., 'Human studies with probiotics and prebiotics: Clinical implications', *British Journal of Nutrition* 2002;87:S241–S246.

Sanders M.E., 'Considerations for use of probiotic bacteria to modulate human health', *Journal of Nutrition* 2000;130:384S–90S.

Sanders M.E., 'Gut flora and the impact of probiotics on human health. Notes taken from Symposium in conjunction with American College of Gastroenterology', Annual Scientific Meeting 16 October 2007.

Sanders M.E., 'Probiotics: Publication of the Institute of Food Technologists expert panel on food safety and nutrition'. *Food Technology* 1999;53(11):67–77.

Sanders M.E., et al., 'Probiotics: Their potential to impact human health', *Council for Agricultural Science and Technology* (CAST) 2007; Issue Paper no.36. http://www.cast-science.org/

Schauss A.G., et al., 'Phytochemical and nutrient composition of the freeze-dried amazonian palm berry: *Euterpe oleraceae* Mart', *Journal of Agricultural and Food Chemistry* 2006;54(22):8598–603

Simmering R. and Blaut M., 'Pro- and prebiotics: The tasty guardian angels?' *Applied Microbiology & Biotechnology* 2001;55:19–28.

Slavin J.L., 'Dietary fiber and body weight', *Nutrition* 2005;21(3):411–18.

Trinidad T.P., et al., 'Interactive effects of Ca and SOFA on absorption in the distal colon of man', *Nutrition Research* 1993;13:417.

Veldhuijzen I., et al., and EARSS participants, 'European Antimicrobial Resistance Surveillance System (EARSS): Susceptibility testing of invasive *Staphylococcus aureus*', *EuroSurveillance* 2000;5(3):24.

Wynne A.G., et al., 'An *in vitro* assessment of the effects of broad-spectrum antibiotics on the human gut microflora and concomitant isolation of a *Lactobacillus plantarum* with anti-Candida activities', *Anaerobe* 2004;10 (3):165–9.

Part Two

Aas J.A., et al., 'Defining the normal bacterial flora of the oral cavity', *Journal of Clinical Microbiology* 2005;43:5721–32.

Abedon S.T., Biology 114 lecture (Spring 2007 syllabus), Chapter on Antimicrobial Therapy, Ohio State University, 1680 University Drive, Mansfield, OH 44906,

USA. http://www.mansfield.ohio-state.edu/~sabedon/black13.htm

Aiba Y., et al., 'Lactic acid-mediated suppression of *Helicobacter pylori* by the oral administration of *Lactobacillus salivarius* as a probiotic in a gnotobiotic murine model', *American Journal of Gastroenterology* 1998;93:2097–101.

Alvarez-Olmos M.I. and Oberhelman R.A., 'Probiotic agents and infectious diseases: A modern perspective on a traditional therapy', *Clinical Infectious Diseases* 2001;1;32(11):1567–76.

Arunachalam K., et al., 'Enhancement of natural immune function by dietary consumption of *Bifidobacterium lactis*', *European Journal of Clinical Nutrition* 2000;54:263–7.

Barrons R., et al., 'Use of *Lactobacillus* probiotics for bacterial genitourinary infections in women: A review', *Clinical Therapeutics* 2008;30:453–68.

Bartlett J.G., 'Historical perspectives on studies of *Clostridium difficile* and *C. difficile* infection', *Clinical Infectious Diseases* 2008;46(Suppl 1):S4–11.

Blasi F., et al., 'Detection of *Chlamydia pneumoniae* but not *Helicobacter pylori* in atherosclerotic plaques of aortic aneurysms', *Journal of Clinical Microbiology* 1996;34(11):2766–9.

Borody T., 'Flora power: Fecal bacteria cure chronic *C. Difficile* diarrhoea', *American Journal of Gastroenterology* 2000;95(11):3028–9.

Brady L.J., et al., 'The role of probiotic cultures in the prevention of colon cancer', *Journal of Nutrition* 2000;130(2S):410S–14S.

Brinkeborn R.M., et al., 'Echinaforce and other Echinacea fresh plant preparations in the treatment of the common cold', *Phytomedicine* 1999;6(1):1–5.

Burns A.J. and Rowland I.R., 'Anti-carcinogenicity of probiotics and prebiotics', *Current Issues in Intestinal Microbiology* 2000;1(1):13–24.

Burton J.P., et al. 'Improved understanding of the bacterial vaginal microbiota of women before and after probiotic instillation', *Applied Environmental Microbiology* 2003;69:97–101.

Burton J.P., et al., 'A preliminary study of the effect of probiotic *Streptococcus salivarius* K12 on oral malodour parameters', *Journal of Applied Microbiology* 2006;100:754–64.

Burton J.P., et al., 'Detection of *Atopobium vaginae* in postmenopausal women by cultivation-independent methods warrants further investigation', *Journal of Clinical Microbiology* 2004;42:1829–31.

Burton J.P. and Reid G., 'Evaluation of the bacterial vaginal flora of 20 postmenopausal women by direct (Nugent score) and molecular (polymerase chain reaction and denaturing gradient gel electrophoresis) techniques', *Journal of Infectious Diseases* 2002;186:1770–80.

Callaway, E., 'Superbug "condom" could slow spread of drug resistance', *New Scientist* 19 December 2008; issue 2687.

Campieri M., 'Probiotics in inflammatory bowel disease: New insight to pathogenesis or a possible therapeutic alternative?' *Gastroenterology* 1999;116:1246–9.

Cannon C.P., et al., 'Antibiotic treatment of *Chlamydia pneumoniae* after acute coronary syndrome', *New England Journal of Medicine* 2005;352(16):1646–54.

Carlsson J., et al., 'Early establishment of *Streptococcus salivarius* in the mouth of infants', *Journal of Dental Research* 1970;49:415–18.

Carman R.J., et al., 'Ciprofloxacin at low levels disrupts colonization resistance of human fecal microflora growing in chemostats', Extract, *Regulatory Toxicology and Pharmacology* 2004;40(3):319–26.

Cebra J.J., 'Influences of microbiota on intestinal immune system development', *Journal of Immunology* 1999;69:1046S–51S.

Chadwick V.S., et al., 'Activation of the mucosal immune system in irritable bowel syndrome', *Gastroenterology* 2002;122(7):1778–83.

Cherbut C., et al., 'Acacia Gum is a bifidogenic dietary fibre with high digestive tolerance in healthy humans', *Journal of Microbial Ecology in Health and Disease* 2003;15(1):43–50.

Chiang B.L., et al., 'Enhancing immunity by dietary consumption of a probiotic lactic acid bacterium (*Bifidobacterium lactis HN019*): Optimization and definition of cellular immune responses', *European Journal of Clinical Nutrition* 2000;54:849–55.

Cummings J.H., et al., 'Prebiotic digestion and fermentation', *American Journal of Clinical Nutrition* 2001;73(2):415S–20S.

de Vrese M., et al., 'Effect of *Lactobacillus gasseri* PA 16/8, *Bifidobacterium longum* SP 07/3, *B.bifidum* MF 20/5 on common cold episodes: A double blind, randomized, controlled trial', *Clinical Nutrition* 2005;24(4):481–91.

Dial S., et al., 'Proton pump inhibitor use and risk of community-acquired *Clostridium difficile*-associated disease defined by prescription for oral vancomycin therapy', *Canadian Medical Association Journal* 2006;175:745–8.

Eyssen H., 'Role of gut microflora in metabolism of lipids and sterols', *Proceedings of the Nutrition Society* 1973;32:59–63.

Furrie E., 'Probiotics and allergy', *Proceedings of the Nutrition Society* 2005;64(4):465–9.

Hatakka K., et al., 'Effect of long term consumption of probiotic milk on infections in children attending day care centres: Double blind, randomised trial', *British Medical Journal* 2001;322:1–5.

Gibson G.R., 'Fibre and effects on probiotics (the prebiotic concept)', *Clinical Nutrition Supplements* 2004;1(2):25–31.

Gill H.S., 'Probiotics to enhance anti-infective defences in the gastrointestinal tract', *Best Practice Research Clinical Gastroenterology* 2003;17:755–73.

Glaser A., 'Groups ask FDA to ban antibacterial products containing triclosan: Beyond pesticides/national coalition against the misuse of pesticides', *Pesticides and You* 2005;25(3):18.

Goldin B.R. and Gorbach S.L., et al., 'Alterations of the intestinal microflora by diet, oral antibiotics and *Lactobacillus*: Decreased production of free amines from aromatic nitro compounds, azo dyes and glucuronides', *Journal of the National Cancer Institute* 1984:73;689–95.

Hanson L.A., 'Protective effects of breast-feeding against urinary tract infection', *Acta Pædiatrica* 2004;93:154–6.

Hickson M., et al., 'Use of probiotic *Lactobacillus* preparation to prevent diarrhoea associated with antibiotics: Randomized double blind placebo controlled trial', *British Medical Journal* 2007;335(7610):80.

Hilton E., et al., 'Ingestion of yogurt containing *Lactobacillus acidophilus* as prophylaxis for candidal vaginitis', *Annals of Internal Medicine* 1992;116(5):353–7.

Huang J.S., et al., 'Efficacy of probiotic use in acute diarrhea in children', *Digestive Diseases and Sciences* 2002;47:2625–34.

Hutchins A., 'Flaxseed influences urinary lignan excretion in a dose-dependent manner in postmenopausal women', *Cancer Epidemiology Biomarkers & Prevention* 2000;9:1113–18.

Imase K., et al., 'Lactobacillus reuteri tablets suppress Helicobacter pylori infection: A double-blind randomised placebo-controlled cross-over clinical study', Kansenshogaku Zasshi 2007;81:387–93.

Ivory K., et al., 'Oral delivery of Lactobacillus casei Shirota modifies allergen-induced immune responses in allergic rhinitis', Clinical and Experimental Allergy 2008;38(8):1282–9.

Jackson L.A., et al., 'Isolation of Chlamydia pneumoniae from a carotid endarterectomy specimen', Journal of Infectious Diseases 1997;176(1): 292–5.

Jacobs, G., Beat Candida Through Diet: A Complete Dietary Programme for Sufferers of Candidiasis, Trafalgar, 1997.

Kendrick M., The Great Cholesterol Con, Blake Publishing, 2008.

King T.S., et al., 'Abnormal colonic fermentation in irritable bowel syndrome', Lancet 1998;352:1187–9.

Marshall B.J., 'Helicobacter pylori', American Journal of Gastroenterology 1994;89:S116–S28.

Marteau P., 'A probiotic-vitamin combination to protect against common cold', Clinical Nutrition 2005;24(4):479–80.

Mathern J. and Verbruggen M., 'Special report: Flax lignans', Total Health 2003:1–15.

Matsen J., The Secrets to Great Health, Goodwin Books, 1998.

McDonald L., 'Clostridium difficile responding to a new threat from an old enemy', Infection Control and Hospital Epidemiology 2005;26(8):672–5.

McFarland L.V. and Dublin S., 'Meta-analysis of probiotics for the treatment of irritable bowel syndrome', World Journal of Gastroenterology 2008;14:2650–61.

Murch S.H., 'Probiotics as mainstream allergy therapy?', Archives of Disease of Childhood 2005; 90(9):881–2.

Myllyluoma E., et al., 'Probiotic supplementation improves tolerance to Helicobacter pylori eradication therapy: A placebo-controlled, double-blind randomized pilot study', Alimentary Pharmacology and Therapeutics 2005;21:1263–72.

Niv E., et al., 'The efficacy of Lactobacillus reuteri ATCC 55730 in the treatment of patients with irritable bowel syndrome: A double blind, placebo-controlled, randomized study', Clinical Nutrition 2005;24(6):925–31.

Nobaek S., et al., 'Alteration of intestinal microflora is associated with reduction in abdominal bloating and pain in patients with irritable bowel syndrome', American Journal of Gastroenterology 2000;95(5):1231–8.

Nomoto K., 'Prevention of infection by probiotics', Journal of Bioscience and Bioengineering 2005;100(6):583–92.

Noverr M.C. and Huffnagle G.B., 'The microflora hypothesis of allergic diseases', Clinical and Experimental Allergy 2005;35:1511.

Oksanen P.J., et al., 'Prevention of travelers diarrhea by Lactobacillus GG', Annals of Medicine 1990;22:53–6.

Olivares M., et al., 'Oral intake of Lactobacillus fermentum CECT5716 enhances the effects of influenza vaccination', Nutrition 2007;23(3):254–60.

Orrhage K., et al., 'Effect of supplements with Bifidobacterium longum and Lactobacillus acidophilus on the intestinal microbiota during administration of clindamycin', Microbial Ecology in Health and Disease 1994;7:17–25.

O'Sullivan M.A. and O'Morain C.A., 'Bacterial supplementation in the irritable bowel syndrome: A randomized double-blind placebo-controlled crossover study', Digestive & Liver Diseases 2000;32(4):294–301.

Ouwehand A.C., et al., 'Differences in *Bifidobacterium* flora composition in allergic and healthy infants', *Journal of Allergy and Clinical Immunology* 2001;108:144–5.

Park S.K., et al., 'The effect of probiotics on *Helicobacter pylori* eradication', *Hepatogastroenterology* 2007;54:2032–6.

Parvez S., et al., 'Probiotics and their fermented food products are beneficial for health', *Journal of Applied Microbiology* 2006;100(6):1171–85.

Paterson D, et al., 'Putting back the bugs: Bacterial treatment relieves chronic diarrhoea', *Medical Journal of Australia* 1994;160(4):232–3.

Pelto L., et al., '*Lactobacillus* GG modulates milk-induced immune inflammatory response in milk-hypersensitive adults', *Nutrition Today* 1996;Suppl.31:45S–46S.

Pelto L., et al., 'Probiotic bacteria down-regulate the milk-induced inflammatory response in milk-hypersensitive subjects but have an immunostimulatory effect in healthy subjects', *Clinical and Experimental Allergy* 1998;28:1474–9.

Penders J., et al., 'The role of the intestinal microbiota in the development of atopic disorders', *Allergy* 2007;62(11):1223–36.

Peng G.C., et al., 'The efficacy and safety of heat killed *Lactobacillus paracasei* for the treatment of perennial allergic rhinitis induced by house dust mite', *Paediatric Allergy and Immunology* 2005;16:433.

Pereira D.I. and Gibson G.R., 'Effects of consumption of probiotics and prebiotics on serum lipid levels in humans', *Critical Reviews in Biochemical and Molecular Biology* 2002;37:259–81.

Pierce P.F. et al., 'Antibiotic-associated pseudomembranous colitis: An epidemiologic investigation of a cluster of cases', *Journal of Infectious Diseases* 1982;145:269–74.

Pirotta M., et al., 'Effect of *Lactobacillus* in preventing post-antibiotic vulvovaginal candidiasis: A randomised controlled trial', *British Medical Journal* 2004;329:548.

Pitkala K.H., et al., 'Fermented cereal with *specific bifidobacteria* normalizes bowel movements in elderly nursing home residents: A randomized, controlled trial', *Journal of Nutrition Health and Aging* 2007;11:305–11.

Plummer S.F., et al., '*Clostridium difficile* pilot study: Effects of probiotic supplementation on the incidence of *C. difficile* diarrhoea', *International Microbiology* 2004;7(1):59–62.

Plummer S.F., et al., 'Effects of probiotics on the composition of the intestinal microbiota following antibiotic therapy', *International Journal of Antimicrobial Agents* 2005;26(1):69–74.

Posserud I., et al., 'Small intestinal bacterial overgrowth in patients with irritable bowel syndrome', *Gut* 2007;56(6):802–8.

Prasad K., 'Dietary flax seed in prevention of hypercholesterolemic atherosclerosis, *Atherosclerosis* 1997;132:69–76.

Prescott S.L. and Björkstén B., 'Probiotics for the prevention or treatment of allergic diseases', *Journal of Allergy and Clinical Immunology* 2007;120(2):255–62.

Quinlan A., 'MRSA faces defeat from wild flower', *Irish Examiner* 16 November 2007.

Rafter J., 'The effects of probiotics on colon cancer development', *Nutrition Research Reviews* 2004;17:277–84.

Rahimi R., et al., 'A meta-analysis on the efficacy of probiotics for maintenance of remission and prevention of clinical and endoscopic relapse in Crohn's disease', *Digestive Diseases and Sciences* 2008;53(5):1278–84.

Ravnskov U., *The Cholesterol Myths: Exposing the Fallacy that Saturated Fat and*

Cholesterol Cause Heart Disease, New Trends Publishing, 2001.

Reddy G.V., et al., 'Antitumour activity of yogurt components', *Journal of Food Protection* 1983;46:8–11.

Reid G. and Bocking A., 'The potential for probiotics to prevent bacterial vaginosis and preterm labor', *American Journal of Obstetrics and Gynecology* 2003; 189(4):1202–8.

Reid G., et al., 'Oral Probiotics Can Resolve Urogenital Infections', *FEMS Immunology and Medical Microbiology* 2001;30(1):49–52.

Reid G., et al., 'Oral use of *Lactobacillus rhamnosus* GR-1 and *L. fermentum* RC-14 significantly alters vaginal flora: Randomized, placebo-controlled trial in 64 healthy women', *FEMS Immunology and Medical Microbiology* 2003;35:131–4.

Reid G., 'Probiotic Agents to Protect the Urogenital Tract Against Infection', *American Journal of Clinical Nutrition* 2001;73(2):437S–43S.

Reid G., 'Probiotics in the treatment of diarrheal diseases', *Current Infectious Disease Reports* 2000;2(1):78.

Reid G., 'The importance of guidelines in the development and application of probiotics', *Current Pharmaceutical Design* 2005;11:11–16.

Ritchie M., et al., 'Adaptive immunomodulation resulting from Echinaforce', Poster presentation. Phytopharmaka and Phytotherapie Kongress; 14–16 February 2008, Berlin, Germany.

Rosenberg M., 'The science of bad breath', *Scientific American* 2002;286:72–9.

Rubaltelli F.F., 'Intestinal flora in breast- and bottle-fed infants', *Journal of Perinatal Medicine* 1998;26:186–91.

Saavedra J.M., et al., 'Feeding of *Bifidobacterium bifidum* and *Streptococcus thermophilus* to infants in hospital for prevention of diarrhoea and shedding of rotavirus', *Lancet* 1994;344:1046–9.

Saggiro A., 'Probiotics in the treatment of irritable bowel syndrome', *Journal of Clinical Gastroenterology* 2004;38(II):S104–6.

Saikali J., 'Fermented milks, probiotic cultures, and colon cancer', *Nutrition and Cancer* 2004;49:14–24.

Singh J., et al., '*Bifidobacterium longum*, a lactic acid-producing intestinal bacterium inhibits colon cancer and modulates the intermediate biomarkers of colon carcinogenesis', *Carcinogenesis* 1997;18:833–41.

Soulsby E.J., 'Resistance to antimicrobials in humans and animals', *British Medical Journal* 2005;331(7527):1219–20.

Strachan D.P., 'Hayfever, hygiene and household size', *British Medical Journal* 1989;299:1259.

Suarez F.L., et al., 'The treatment of lactose intolerance', *Alimentary Pharmacology and Therapeutics* 1995;9:589–97.

Tagg J.R., 'Prevention of streptococcal pharyngitis by anti-*Streptococcus pyogenes* bacteriocin-like inhibitory substances (BLIS) produced by *Streptococcus salivarius*', *Indian Journal of Medical Research* 2004;119S:13–16.

Tannock G.W., 'The bowel microflora: An important source of urinary tract pathogens', *World Journal of Urology* 1999;17:339–44.

Taper H.S. and Roberfroid M.B., 'Inhibitory effect of dietary inulin or oligofructose on the development of cancer metastases', *Anticancer Research* 2000;20:4291–4.

Taylor G.R.J. and Williams C.M., 'Effects of probiotics and prebiotics on blood lipids', *British Journal of Nutrition* 1998;80(1):S225–30.

Trinidad T.P., et al., 'Interactive effects of Ca and SOFA on absorption in the distal colon of man', *Nutrition Research* 1993;13:417.

Tubelius P., et al., 'Increasing work-place healthiness with the probiotic *Lactobacillus reuteri*: A randomised, double-blind placebo-controlled study', *Environmental Health* 2005;4:25.

Tungland B.C. and Meyer D., 'Nondigestible oligo- and polysaccharides (dietary fiber): Their physiology and role in human health and food', *Comprehensive Reviews in Food Science and Food Safety* 2002;1:73–92.

Turchet P., et al., 'Effect of fermented milk containing the probiotic *Lactobacillus casei* DN-114001 on winter infections in free-living elderly subjects: A randomised, controlled pilot study', *Journal of Nutrition, Health and Aging* 2003;7(2):75–7.

Van Loo J., et al., 'The SYNCAN project: Goals, set-up, first results and settings of the human intervention study', *British Journal of Nutrition* 2005;93:S91–8.

Viljanen M., et al., 'Probiotics in the treatment of atopic eczema/dermatitis syndrome in infants: A double-blind placebo-controlled trial', *Allergy* 2005;60:494–500.

Weizman Z., et al., 'Effect of a probiotic infant formula on infections in child care centers: Comparison of two probiotic agents', *Pediatrics* 2005;115:5–9.

Wilhelm S.M., et al., 'Effectiveness of probiotics in the treatment of irritable bowel syndrome', *Pharmacotherapy* 2008;28:496–505.

Wilkinson E.G., et al., 'Treatment of periodontal and other soft tissue diseases of the oral cavity with coenzyme Q10', *Biomedical and Clinical Aspects of CoQ10* 1977;1:251–6.

Winkler P., et al., 'Effect of a dietary supplement containing probiotic bacteria plus vitamins and minerals on common cold infections and cellular immune parameters', *International Journal of Clinical Pharmacology, Therapy and Toxicology* 2005;43:318–26.

Woelkart K., et al., 'Bioavailability and pharmacokinetics of Echinacea purpurea preparations and their interaction with the immune system', *International Journal of Clinical Pharmacology and Therapeutics* 2006;44(9):401–8.

Wollowski I., et al., 'Protective role of probiotics and prebiotics in colon cancer', *American Journal of Clinical Nutrition* 2001;73(2 Suppl):451S–5S.

Yang H.B., et al., 'Pretreatment with *Lactobacillus*- and *Bifidobacterium*-containing yogurt can improve the efficacy of quadruple therapy in eradicating residual *Helicobacter pylori* infection after failed triple therapy', *American Journal of Clinical Nutrition* 2006;83:864–9.

Young E., et al., 'A population study of food intolerance', *Lancet* 1994;343:127–9.

Part Three

'Joint FAO/WHO Food Standards Programme. Codex Committee on Food Labelling', *Codex Alimentarius Commission* 30th Session, 6–10 May 2002, http://www.codexalimentarius.net/web/index_en.jsp

'Joint FAO/WHO Expert Consultation: Report of the Joint Food and Agriculture Organization (FAO) of the United Nations/World Health Organization (WHO) Expert Consultation on Evaluation of Health and Nutritional Properties of Probiotics in Food Including Powder Milk with Live Lactic Acid Bacteria', *Codex Alimentarius Commission*, http://www.who.int/foodsafety/publications/fs_management/en/probiotics.pdf

'Report of the Joint WHO/FAO Expert Consultation: Diet, nutrition and the prevention of chronic diseases', WHO Technical Report Series TRS 2003.

'Probiotic Food Supplements: Best Practice Standard', August 2006, published by the Health Food Manufacturers' Association, 1 Wolsey Road, East Molesey, Surrey KT8 9EL, telephone: 0208 481 7100, http://www.hfma.co.uk/probiotics.asp

European Commission MEM0/03/188, 'The proposed regulation on health & nutrition claims: Myths & misunderstandings', Issued Brussels, 1 October 2003.

European Commission, Press Release (IP/08/37), 'Novel Foods', 14 January 2008.

European Commission, Council Minutes (5509/08) 'Claims: Nutrition and health claims made on foods', extract from the minutes of the 2843rd Council meeting (Agriculture and Fisheries) of 21 January 2008.

Articles 10–19 of the EU Nutrition and Health Claims Regulation.

Regulation (EC) no 1924/2006 of the European Parliament and of The Council on Nutrition and Health claims made on foods, 20 December 2006.

European Food Safety Authority, 'Additional information relating to health and nutrition claims', www.efsa.europa.eu

UK Food Standards Agency, Table 3 – Probiotic Ingredients, Protein and Vitamins, www.food.gov.uk

Adams M.R. and Marteau P., 'On the safety of lactic acid bacteria from food', *International Journal of Food Microbiology* 1995;27:263–4.

Alberda C., et al., 'Effects of probiotic therapy in critically ill patients: A randomized, double-blind, placebo-controlled trial', *American Journal of Clinical Nutrition* 2007;85:816–23.

Besselink M.G.H., et al., 'Probiotic prophylaxis in predicted severe acute pancreatitis: A randomized, double-blind, placebo-controlled trial', *Lancet* 2008;371(9613):651–9.

Borriello SP, et al., 'Safety of probiotics that contain *lactobacilli* or *bifidobacteria*'. *Clinical Infectious Diseases* 2003;36:775–80.

Ishibashi N., et al., 'Probiotics and Safety', *American Journal of Clinical Nutrition* 2001;73(2):465S–70S.

Mangiante G., et al., '*Lactobacillus plantarum* reduces infection of pancreatic necrosis in experimental acute pancreatitis', *Digestive Surgery* 2001;18(1):47–50.

Marteau P., 'Tolerance of probiotics and prebiotics', *Journal of Clinical Gastroenterology* 2004;38(6 Suppl):S67–9.

Rayes N., et al., 'Supply of pre- and probiotics reduces bacterial infection rates after liver transplantation: A randomized, double-blind trial', *American Journal of Transplantation* 2005;5:125–30.

Reid G., et al., 'Potential uses of probiotics in clinical practice', *Clinical Microbiology Reviews* 2003;16:658–72.

Salminen S., et al., 'Demonstration of safety of probiotics: A review', *International Journal of Food Microbiology* 1998;44(1–2):93–106.

Sanders M.E., 'Probiotics: Strains matter', *Functional Foods & Nutraceuticals Magazine*, June 2007:36–41.

Wolf B.W., et al., 'Safety and tolerance of *Lactobacillus reuteri* supplementation to a population infected with the human immunodeficiency virus', *Food and Chemical Toxicology* 1998;36:1085–94.

Index

elderly people (*cont.*)
  oral health, 168
elecampane, 134
emergency action plan, 142–6
Enterococci, 131, 239
enzymes, 28, 38, 43, 85, 124
epiglottis, 60
erythromycin, 113
Escherichia coli, 24, 31, 62, 63, 66, 67, 72,
    106, 119, 131–2, 210, 236, 239
espelta, 45
exercise, 41, 208

faeces, *see* stools
FAP (familial adenomatous polyposis), 193
fats, 63, 177, 182
  polyunsaturated, 51, 182
  see also hydrogenated fats and oils
fatty acids, 28
  omega-3, 72, 161, 253
  omega-6, 161
  short-chain (SCFAs), 78, 251–2
  trans- (TFAs), 177–8, 180
fermentation, 74, 77, 80, 91, 181, 214
fermented foods, 80–7, 220
  list of active foods, 85–6
fibre, 44, 45–6, 64, 70, 72, 74, 88–104,
    143, 184, 196
  benefits, 91–2
  and bowel movement, 202, 206–7
  insoluble and soluble, 89–91
  list of food sources, 103–4
  mucilaginous, 46
  recommended amounts, 92
  resistant starch, 90, 91
  supplements, 99–100
  warning, 102–3
fibrinogen, 179, 185
fibromyalgia, 214, 258
Fischer, Martin Henry, 105
fish, 196, 252–3
flatulence, *see* gas
flavonoid supplements, 224, 235
flax fibre, 216, 253
flaxseed, 46, 95–9, 122, 143–4, 184
  not advised for toddlers, 102
Fleming, Alexander, 106, 107, 124
Florey, Howard, 107
flu, 187–91, 260
folic acid, 87, 180
food
  chewing, 38–9, 60, 142–3, 171, 216, 224
  diary, 216
  eating out, 39, 55

functional, 71–2
  low-fat packaged, 51, 55, 146, 182
  mealtimes, 38–40, 142–3
  processed, 55, 145, 177, 197, 259
  sensitivity and allergies, 57, 156, 159,
    213, 214, 215
  spicy, 43, 171
  temperature, 43
  washing and preparing, 119–20
  see also diet; fibre; prebiotics
Food and Agriculture Organization of the
    United Nations, 21, 32, 71, 226
FOS (fructo-oligosaccharides), 52, 77, 78,
    217, 280
Framingham Heart Study, 176
fried food, 51
fructose, malabsorption of, 214, 216
fruit, 42–3, 45–6, 51, 52, 75, 95, 100, 101,
    112, 144–5, 184, 197, 252, 259
  washing, 119
fruit juices, 43, 52, 89, 101, 145, 191, 212,
    252
fungal infections, 246, 249, 280

garlic, 134, 137, 138, 189, 224, 248
gas, 28, 43, 66, 76–7, 84, 93, 165, 213,
    214, 215, 216, 269, 280
Giardia lamblia, 63, 86
Gibson, Glenn, 71
gingivitis, 171
ginkgo biloba, 161
glucose, *see* blood glucose levels
glyconutrients, 170, 236–7
GORD (gastro-oesophageal reflux disease),
    135
gout, 79
Gratia, André, 107
gullet (oesophagus), 60, 221
gum disease, 58, 165–6, 168, 170, 171, 181
gut (gastrointestinal tract), 57–67
  mucosal lining, 64
  wall, 56, 57, 58, 244–5, 250

H. pylori, see *Helicobacter pylori*
H2 receptor antagonists, 135, 225
haemorrhoids, 84, 89, 95, 98, 200, 203,
    205, 242
halitosis, *see* breath, bad
hand washing, 118–19, 136, 137, 138, 139,
    157, 190
hay fever, 156–7
HCl, *see* hydrochloric acid
healing crisis, 269
heart disease, 89, 96, 145, 176–7, 178–81